REVIEW OF SPECIALIST CHILDREN'S

SERVICES

May 1993

London: HMSO

9308184

CHILD HEALTH SERVICES
LONDON

WX 150

WS 27

Contents

List of figures and tables

Section 1:   The purpose of this review

Contents of this section

1.1: Introduction

This review of specialist children's services in London has been produced at the request of the London Implementation Group. It was commissioned in February 1993 in response to the **Report of the inquiry into London's health services**, also known as the Tomlinson report.

The Tomlinson report pointed out that there is currently widespread duplication of specialist services in London. In its response to this report, entitled **Making London better**, the Government took the view that duplication is not cost effective and might work against maintaining the standards of excellence for which some of these services are internationally recognised.

A series of reviews was commissioned to determine the best way of providing some of these specialist services in the future, and to reduce unnecessary duplication where possible. Six specialist services were chosen: cardiac services, cancer services, neurosciences, renal services, plastic surgery, and specialist children's services. The reviews have been carried out by small groups of experts, each jointly led by an eminent clinician from outside London and a senior NHS manager of a purchasing authority.

Each review group was asked to assess the current and projected needs for a particular specialist service, to define appropriate models of care and criteria for tertiary centres, and to develop a service specification.

The authors of this report were asked to recommend an appropriate pattern of service for specialist children's services, and to suggest where the services should be located to achieve the best clinical outcome.

Specialist Children's Services Review Group
May 1993

1.2: Membership of the Specialist Children's Services Review Group

Chairman
Professor Sir David Hull, Professor of the Department of Child Health, Queen's Medical Centre, Nottingham

Dr Robert F Cooper, Director of Public Health, Solihull Health Authority

Mrs Ann Craft, Director of Nursing, Royal Victoria Infirmary and Associated Hospitals NHS Trust

Dr Zarrina Kurtz, Consultant in Public Health Medicine, South West Thames Regional Health Authority

Professor David Lloyd, Consultant paediatric surgeon, Alderhey Hospital, Liverpool

Lady Jean Lovell-Davies

Dr Roderick MacFaul, Consultant paediatrician, Pinderfields Hospital, Wakefield

Dr Peter Morris, Consultant anaesthetist, Salford Hospital, Manchester

Dr John Oldham, General practitioner, Glossop

Martin W Roberts, Chief executive, Wandsworth Health Authority

Acknowledgements

The Specialist Children's Services Review Group would like to thank all the parents' groups, voluntary and charitable organisations, specialty groups, community health councils, provider units and regional health authorities who contributed to this review. We are particularly grateful for the efforts they made to meet the deadlines imposed by our very tight timetable. We would also like to place on record our appreciation of the invaluable work of Ms Tracy Dighton and, in particular, Miss Ann Ziegler. We are grateful to the Audit Commission for giving us access to unpublished parts of its report, **Children first.**

1.3: **Terms of reference**

The detailed terms of reference given to the Specialist Children's Services Review Group were as follows:

1. To review the literature relating to the organisation and financing of the specialty, with particular regard to studies of services in London.

2. To assess the opportunities for prevention and the need for treatment for the diseases covered by the specialty, and to incorporate views on the developments likely to result from research initiatives, demographic trends and changes in the incidence or prevalence of the diseases.

3. To define appropriate models of care for patients at home and in outpatient departments, day care facilities, hospitals, hospices and hotels, covering all stages of disease, including the management of long-term disability.

4. To define within the above framework the criteria for a multi-disciplinary tertiary centre and to specify the services that should be provided by such a centre.

   To specify the contribution to a multi-disciplinary tertiary centre of individual departments and of other departments on the same hospital site that are not part of the centre itself.

6. To describe the contribution the tertiary centre would make to the teaching of undergraduate and postgraduate students and the requirements necessary for a research base.

7. To comment on the accessibility of services and related issues such as travelling times for patients and their families, and communication issues relating to the burden of care the family will carry.

8. To consider the arrangements necessary to collaborate with local authority social services departments and voluntary agencies.

9. To analyse the services currently available in London; the volume and quality of the workload, and its geographical distribution.

10. To weigh up all these considerations and such other information or advice as is deemed appropriate and to devise a set of proposals for the delivery of care in London, with particular regard to the critical mass that optimises clinical performance.

11. To submit a report to the London Implementation Group by 31 May 1993.

1.4: A note on terminology

Throughout this report we refer to **primary**, **secondary** and **tertiary** services, primary, secondary and tertiary **levels** of care, and the **interfaces** between them. It is important that the meaning of these terms in the context of this report is clearly understood.

Primary care would generally be given by professional staff to whom the patient could refer themselves directly, in particular the general practitioner but also including other professional staff working in the community, such as the practice nurse, health visitor or district nurse. Whilst primary care services are developing in inner cities, some primary care is provided by the community child health medical officers.

Secondary care work for children is that not usually undertaken by general practitioners but is referred by them to a consultant.

Tertiary care is more specialist care or treatment given by a consultant generally after referral from another consultant.

Another way of looking at it is the level of specialist skill required to deal with a particular condition (some of which are rare or complex) in the population at large. What does not define primary, secondary and tertiary care is the location in which it is undertaken. Both secondary and tertiary care can be provided away from the main diagnostic and treatment centre, for example the majority of patients suffering from chronic renal failure can have their dialysis undertaken at home. The point is that the technician and nurse who visit and support them are highly specialised people.

With a shared management protocol, some of these skills are developed by staff members of the primary and secondary care teams by giving them the appropriate expertise to undertake certain treatments normally given by staff in the tertiary centres but with support from them.

1.5: The scope of the review

Specialist tertiary services for children fall into two categories: those that can be defined by the system, organ or disease to which they relate, and those that can be defined by the type of care they provide.

The first category covers cancer services, cardiology and cardiothoracic services, neurology and neurosurgical services, nephrology and urology, endocrinology, gastroenterology, metabolic disease, haematology, infectious diseases, respiratory medicine, immunology and rheumatology.

The second category covers paediatric intensive care, neonatal intensive care, paediatric surgery and other specialist surgery for children.

We felt unable to provide a comprehensive report on all these services within the timetable specified in **Making London better.**(1)   Instead, we elected to concentrate on tertiary services for children in the five areas being covered in the adult specialty reviews, i.e., **cardiothoracic services, renal services, cancer services, plastic surgery,** and **neurosciences.**

We learnt from our colleagues in the Plastic Surgery Review Group that much of the work in plastic surgery was carried out at a secondary level, and therefore we did not give this specialty the same consideration as the others.

Furthermore, it was impossible in the time available to say anything about the condition of the estate, to draw any conclusions about current contract prices, or to make statements about manpower issues.

1.6:   Method of working

Members of the Review Group visited personally as many hospitals and service providers as possible and invited written comments from a wide range of other interested organisations and institutions (to which we received over 100 replies). We also met with a large number of consumer groups, voluntary organisations, community health councils, general practitioner fund-holders, nurses, regional directors of public health and purchasing authorities.

References

1. Department of Health, **Making London better,** London, 1993

Section 2:   Demography

Contents of this section

2.1: The area covered by this review

This review is primarily concerned with specialist services for children in the inner London districts covered by the four Thames health regions. According to the 1991 census, the total adult and child population of the inner London districts is 2.5 million. A breakdown of the child population by age group and region is given in table 1 at the end of this section. Further information on population is given in Appendix 1 and this includes percentage heads of households from the new commonwealth and Pakistan and population density.

For the purposes of this review, "inner London" is defined as the area covered by the following district health authorities:

Bloomsbury and Islington	Newham
Camberwell	Parkside
City and Hackney	Riverside
Hampstead	Tower Hamlets
Lewisham and North	Wandsworth
Southwark	West Lambeth

This is the same definition of inner London used in the **Report of the inquiry into London's health services**, with the exception of Haringey.*

The locations of all the hospitals referred to in this report are shown on the map in figure 1 at the end of this section.

2.2: Assessing relative levels of deprivation**

We assessed the relative levels of deprivation by examining the Townsend deprivation scores for each district. Unfortunately, 1991 based census information for the relevant indicators was not available to the Review Group so estimates derive from the 1981 census were used. Townsend deprivation scores are made up of four factors:

- The percentage of households that are not owner-occupied.
- Unemployment rates.
- Over-crowding in housing.
- The percentage of households who do not own a car.

---

*We have excluded Haringey because there is no hospital of direct relevance to tertiary services for children located within it.

**This review deals with children's needs for specialist services. We agreed that the needs of adolescents would not be covered. The information we gathered therefore relates only to those children aged 14 and under.

Townsend scores for the inner London districts with standardised access ratios[*] to hospital services for children aged 0-14 are shown in Table 2 at the end of this section. Positive scores indicate relative deprivation; scores above 5 are consistent with inner city deprivation. A standardised access ratio over 100 indicates relatively high numbers of episodes of hospital care for a district population compared with the average for the four Thames regions after accounting for any differences in the age and sex structure of the district. (For example, a value of 120 would indicate that, on average, and after accounting for age and sex, children in that district have 20% more actual episodes of hospital care than the average in the four Thames regions as a whole.)

The figures in table 2 show that the inner London populations are relatively deprived, and that children aged 0-14 in inner London have relatively more episodes of inpatient care than children elsewhere in the four Thames regions.

As might be expected, there is a correlation between deprivation and high admission rates to hospital for children aged 0-14. However, evidence from elsewhere indicates that for very high Townsend scores the standardised access ratio dips, which suggests that such populations might experience difficulties in gaining access to health care — see Figure 2 at the end of this section. **Purchasers and providers will need to consider this feature when developing services for inner London in future.**

2.3:   The full range of child health services

It was not part of our terms of reference to make recommendations about secondary level services. However, as we have taken the view that tertiary services should be sited only at hospitals that can provide a full range of child health services at secondary level we have had to make judgements about the long-term viability of these hospitals. There are currently 18 hospital sites with inpatient facilities for children in inner London.

The relatively high use of hospital services by deprived populations would suggest that the population base for a hospital providing a full range of child health services in a depressed area of inner London would be smaller than the average for the country as a whole. **In the light of these considerations, we concluded that for inner London as a whole there could be 8-10 inpatient hospitals, each providing a full range of child health services.**

---

[*] A standardised access ratio is a measure of inpatient activity using the indirect standardisation based on comparison with reference activity levels of the combined four Thames RHA's data. The SAR is standardised for age (0, 1-4, 5-14 bands) and sex. The actual observed episodes of inpatient care for each district's residents are compared with the 'expected' number derived by applying four Thames Regional rates to each of the local districts' populations.

Ambulatory care services provided locally by the main inpatient hospitals would ensure that all children had access to a full range of child health services, no matter where they lived in inner London.

2.4: Access to secondary level services

We commissioned a study of travelling times by public transport to general paediatric services at secondary level. For the purposes of this study we included all hospitals with paediatric services within the boundaries of the M25 motorway — see Figure 3 at the end of this section.

The study revealed that it would take over 50 minutes by public transport for 10% of the population **even within the boundaries of the M25** to reach a hospital with paediatric services.

These findings suggest that some purchasers should review the requirements of their local populations for ambulatory care services.

The findings also warn against the automatic assumption that the current location of secondary level paediatric services will always be the most convenient location for tertiary outreach and shared care services.

References

1. Sir Bernard Tomlinson, **Report of the inquiry into London's health service, medical education and research**, HMSO, London, 1992

Child population in the four Thames Regions
(provisional rebased mid 1991 estimates)

Table 1

Age Group (yrs)	Regions				
	NW	**NE**	**SE**	**SW**	
	No. (%)	No. (%)	No. (%)	No. (%)	Total
<1	51,671 (7.8%)	56,800 (7.8%)	51,400 (7.5%)	40,100 (7.5%)	199,971 (7.7%)
1 - 4	189,754 (28.6%)	210,900 (28.9%)	198,100 (28.9%)	152,700 (28.5%)	751,454 (28.8%)
5 -14	422,343 (63.6%)	461,700 (63.3%)	435,403 (63.6%)	343,100 (64%)	1,662,543 (63.6%)
Total	663,768 (100%)	729,400 (100%)	684,900 (100%)	535,900 (100%)	2,613,968 (100%)
Children under 15 years of age make up: Region	18.6%	19.4%	18.6%	17.7% of the total population of each respectively	
Regional Total Population	3,560,427	3,757,300	3,684,900	3,023,400	14,026,027
Births in 1991	51,459	57,059	51,412	39,975	
Total period fertility rate*	1.82	1.93	1.89	1.82	

* Total period fertility rate: Average number of live births that would occur per woman resident in an area, if women experienced the area's current age-specific fertility rates throughout their childbearing life span.

Figure 1

MAIN CENTRES
Children

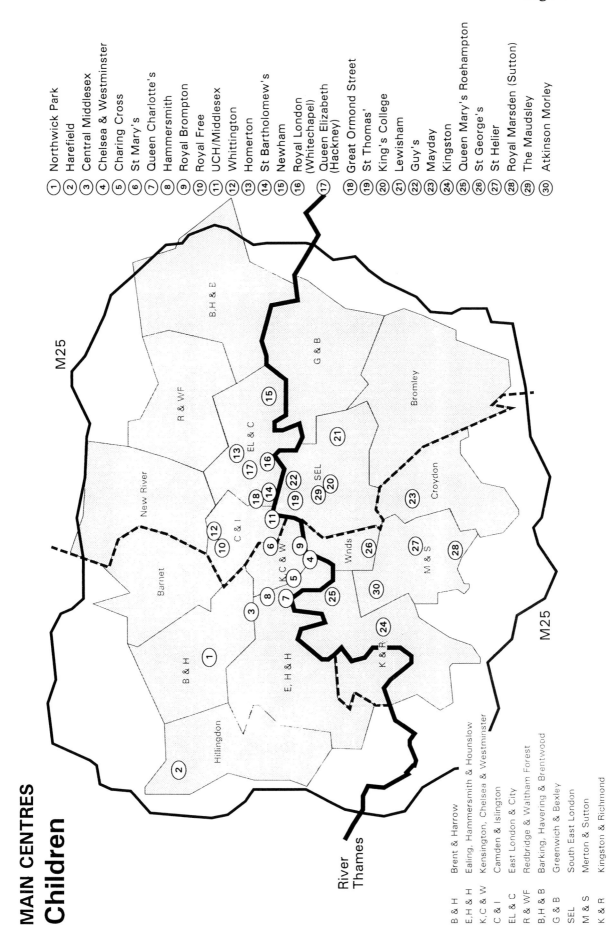

1. Northwick Park
2. Harefield
3. Central Middlesex
4. Chelsea & Westminster
5. Charing Cross
6. St Mary's
7. Queen Charlotte's
8. Hammersmith
9. Royal Brompton
10. Royal Free
11. UCH/Middlesex
12. Whittington
13. Homerton
14. St Bartholomew's
15. Newham
16. Royal London (Whitechapel)
17. Queen Elizabeth (Hackney)
18. Great Ormond Street
19. St Thomas'
20. King's College
21. Lewisham
22. Guy's
23. Mayday
24. Kingston
25. Queen Mary's Roehampton
26. St George's
27. St Helier
28. Royal Marsden (Sutton)
29. The Maudsley
30. Atkinson Morley

B & H   Brent & Harrow
E, H & H   Ealing, Hammersmith & Hounslow
K, C & W   Kensington, Chelsea & Westminster
C & I   Camden & Islington
EL & C   East London & City
R & WF   Redbridge & Waltham Forest
B, H & B   Barking, Havering & Brentwood
G & B   Greenwich & Bexley
SEL   South East London
M & S   Merton & Sutton
K & R   Kingston & Richmond

TABLE 2

ANALYSIS OF 1991 CENSUS DATA, DEPRIVATION ESTIMATES USING 1981 DATA AND 1991/92 HOSPITAL ACTIVITY DATA BY DISTRICT OF RESIDENCE

District of Residence	Total Population	Aged 0-14 years	% aged 0-14 years	Townsend Score Deprivation	OVERALL STANDARDISED ACCESS RATIO (SAR)
INNER LONDON DISTRICTS					
Bloomsbury and Islington	242500	42500	18	7	127
Camberwell	218000	43900	20	7	107
City and Hackney	187400	41300	22	10	108
Hampstead	105000	15800	15	6	118
Harringey	207000	39000	19	4	115
Lewisham and North Southwark	327700	63100	19	6	112
Newham	217100	51100	24	6	109
Parkside	432571	76277	18	9	119
Riverside	290507	39155	13	6	102
Tower Hamlets	164900	40200	24	11	113
Wandsworth	191200	29700	16	5	156
West Lambeth	161400	28900	18	7	133
SUM OF INNER LONDON DISTRICTS	2745278	510932	19	7	117
SUM OF OUTER LONDON DISTRICTS	4265417	785206	18	-1	104
SUM OF ALL OTHER DISTRICTS IN FOUR THAMES RHAs	6979332	1286324	18	-3	89

Figure 2

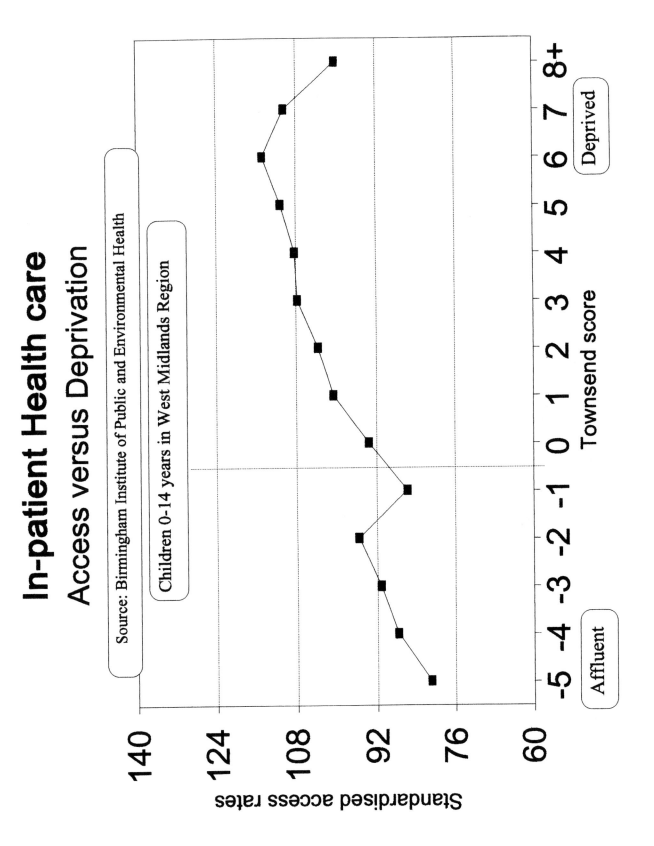

FIGURE 3

SHORTEST TRAVEL TIME BY PUBLIC TRANSPORT (ie. BUS, TUBE OR TRAIN) TO A PAEDIATRIC FACILITY
(Traffic zones in the GLTS area with the London boundary superimposed)

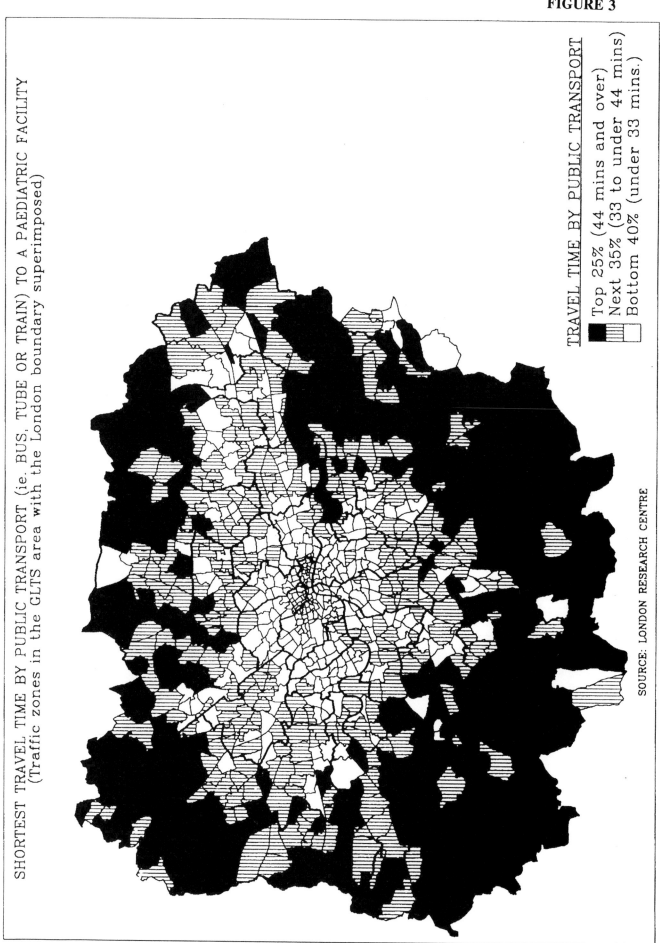

TRAVEL TIME BY PUBLIC TRANSPORT

■ Top 25% (44 mins and over)
▤ Next 35% (33 to under 44 mins)
□ Bottom 40% (under 33 mins.)

SOURCE: LONDON RESEARCH CENTRE

Section 3:   **Tertiary services for children in London**

Contents of this section

3.1: Factors that have affected the way specialist children's services have developed in London

Special children's hospitals

One hundred years ago, when infectious diseases and malnutrition were the commonest health problems, the sick children of London were admitted to special children's hospitals.

Sited as much for the availability of wet nurses as for the convenience of patients and their families, these hospitals were designed as far as possible to avoid cross-infection, and parents were excluded. Most of them have long since closed.

Specialist services for children

Specialist services for children are a much more recent development. Even though some of the special children's hospitals established close links with nearby medical schools — Paddington Green Hospital with St Mary's, for example — the children were not cared for by specialists, but by ordinary physicians who had an interest in children's diseases. It is only in the last 50 years that consultants who work only with children (paediatricians) have been appointed.

Thirty years ago, many of the senior paediatricians appointed to the London teaching hospitals also had sessions at the Hospital for Sick Children, Great Ormond Street.* These paediatricians, including RC Lightwood at St Mary's Hospital, PR Evans at Guy's Hospital, BE Schlesinger at University College Hospital, and WPH Sheldon at King's College Hospital, tended to transfer to Great Ormond Street Hospital those children with complex or undiagnosed problems. As a result, the hospital began to establish departments for children with special problems and laboratories to investigate diseases of childhood. As the reputation of Great Ormond Street Hospital grew, parents with influence began to request that their children were sent there directly.

Academic departments of child health in the London medical schools

The London medical schools were slow to establish their own academic departments of paediatrics and child health. When these departments were set up, the consultant appointments linking them with Great Ormond Street Hospital were discontinued, and the medical schools developed their own tertiary services. Thus Guy's Hospital developed specialist services for children with renal disorders, and King's College Hospital developed services for children with liver disease.

---

* The Hospital for Sick Children, Great Ormond Street, is commonly referred to simply as "Great Ormond Street Hospital". In order to avoid confusion, we have adopted this title throughout this report.

This meant that non-teaching hospitals gradually had the choice of referring children either to Great Ormond Street Hospital or to the specialist services in the teaching hospitals. However, because of its size and the range of services it offers, the collective clinical skills at Great Ormond Street Hospital have always exceeded those in the individual teaching hospitals. Indeed, many paediatricians in the UK have done some of their post-MRCP training at Great Ormond Street Hospital and the associated University of London Institute of Child Health.

3.2: Factors likely to affect the way specialist children's services will develop in the future

Specialty paediatrics and the care of the "whole" child

While there will always be a need for specialist skills that focus exclusively on each of the body's major systems, it is now generally accepted that such a narrow "perspective of disorder" can create its own problems for the effective management of a sick child and the support of his or her family. Renal failure is not uncommon in children after cardiac surgery; children with severe neurological disorders often experience feeding difficulties; children on modern cytotoxic therapy may need a brief period of intensive care.... What has become separate needs to be brought together again. Furthermore, many of the "new" specialties cover many systems — infectious disease, immune competence, metabolic disorders and nutrition are just a few examples.

Developments in maternity services

Rapid developments in fetal imaging in the last few years mean that many physical abnormalities — defects of the heart, central nervous system, kidney and bowel, for example — can now be identified before a baby is born. There are obvious advantages for children with such defects if pre- and post-natal care — as well as counselling services for the parents — can be provided on the same site.

Distinctions between services for adolescents and services for adults

Happily, the treatment of children with chronic illnesses is becoming increasingly successful. Thus it is rare for children with diabetes to be admitted to hospital or for them to develop complications during childhood; children with cystic fibrosis can now expect to enjoy a normal adult life; and 1 in 2,000 young adults will have been "cured" of a cancer of childhood. These advances mean it is now much easier to distinguish between services that are provided specifically for children and services that are provided for adults.

Clear distinctions are particularly important for two groups: children with disabilities, who need special help to achieve the independence which is a characteristic of adult life, and adolescents, who need a full range of medical services, including specialist services, which acknowledge that they are neither children nor independent adults. It is being increasingly appreciated that it is in the best interests of the patient to ensure that there are stated interfaces between services for children and services for adults.

"Patient-centred" care

Developments in paediatric medicine have been accompanied by a growing awareness that a child's quality of life — and the management of a child's illness — can be greatly improved if the parents and family are able to provide as much of the care themselves within their own home, locality, school and hospital.

3.3:   Why change is needed

Taking all the above factors into account, it is easy to see why the specialist services that have developed in London over the years are not ideally placed to meet the current or future needs of children. There is now widespread agreement between parents and professionals alike that what is needed is a review leading to a number of short-term adjustments and a longer-term strategy.

However, any review of specialist children's services cannot take place in isolation; in addition to the considerations outlined above, it must take into account the recently proposed changes to the pattern of London's health services as a whole, and of the changes in the way health services are funded.

Outside the four main Thames regions, tertiary care services for children are usually provided from a major centre with a full range of paediatric specialty services. Usually, services are located within one city and often, but not invariable, on one site. Where in other cities the paediatric provision is split between hospitals and attempts are made to reduce such division and characteristically, outside the four Thames regions, tertiary services are provided within the framework of one major university paediatric and child health department with its linkages to surgical specialities treating children. Overall, there is a balance more greatly in favour of coordination of tertiary services for children outside the four Thames regions. Within the four Thames regions, however, the situation is much more disparate and fragmented and this is illustrated by reference to Table 3 at the end of this section.

The only comprehensive range of paediatric specialist services is provided at Great Ormond Street Hospital. All other teaching hospital paediatric service departments in the four Thames regions have varying degrees of incomplete tertiary care provision.

The children's specialist review has consequently reviewed the present location and range of tertiary care and paediatatric services and although we have focussed upon the specialties requested by LIG ie, oncology, renal services, neurosciences, plastic and burns and cardiology, it is necessary to consider them within the framework of the other children's tertiary care specialist services.

Changes to the overall pattern of services in London

This review of specialist children's services was initiated in **Making London better**, the Government's response to the 1992 Tomlinson report on London's health services (see section 1.1, above). **Making London better** sets out a strategy for change in London's health services as a whole, and this review was carried out in the context of that strategy. The key elements of the strategy are:

- To develop better local primary and community health services.
- To provide a better-balanced hospital service on fewer sites than at present.
- To streamline specialist services.
- To consolidate medical education and research through a programme of mergers of undergraduate medical schools with multi-faculty colleges of the University of London.

From the proposals set out in **Making London better**, we took particular notice of the following observations and recommendations:

- the reference to consultation on a proposal to close the accident and emergency department at Charing Cross Hospital. (para.56)

- the commitment to retain the accident and emergency department at either University College Hospital or the Middlesex Hospital. (para.57)

- the reference to the future of the accident and emergency department at St Bartholomew's Hospital. (para.58)

- the reference to the consolidation on a single site of the accident and emergency departments at Guy's Hospital and St Thomas's Hospital. (para.59)

- the wish to see further progress towards greater integration of services between University College Hospital and the Middlesex Hospital, Great Ormond Street Hospital and the National Hospital for Neurology and Neurosurgery. (para 66)

- the statement that hospitals in west London "cannot be considered in isolation from each other whether in respect of patient services, education or research." (para 62)

- the proposal that the Queen Elizabeth Hospital, Hackney, should link with the Homerton Hospital (para 74(c))

- the need to consider the services provided at St George's Hospital in conjunction with those at Queen Mary's Hospital, Roehampton, and Kingston Hospital and St Helier Hospital. (para 76)

- that the Government recognised that the specialty reviews might lead to the modification of the general proposals for change to acute services set out in **Making London Better** (para 50)

Making London better also states that the Department of Health will meet the excess costs of the special health authorities in line with the CASPE analysis in 1994/95 (para.88). This proposal will give special health authorities time to plan and move into the market. There is also a reference to the fact that general practitioners and health authorities outside London are already sending fewer patients to London hospitals for treatment (para 99).

Financial considerations

The Tomlinson report makes a number of general observations about funding that are directly relevant to this review of specialist children's services. The report states:

- "Under current formulae, all inner London districts except Tower Hamlets and City and Hackney will lose under full-weighted capitation." (para 84)

- "It is not possible to predict how inner London district health authorities will respond to changes in their capitation." (para 85)

- "The inner London districts will face problems when special health authorities come into the market." (para 88)

Since we concluded that tertiary services should be based at hospitals with a full range of secondary level child health services, we had to consider the possible responses of purchasers in inner London to a loss of financial resources.

Only two of the hospitals listed in table 3 of the Tomlinson report — St George's Hospital and King's College Hospital — have an "exclusive population "of a size approaching that necessary to support a full range of child health services at secondary level". *

There is an urgent need for purchasers throughout the four Thames regions to decide how they are going to ensure a full range of child health services is available to all their residents.

---

* Table 3 can be found on page 29 of the Tomlinson report. How an "exclusive population" is calculated is explained in para.106. The London Inquiry looked at the surrounding area of each of the main acute hospitals in inner London and plotted the isochrones (the boundaries of these areas) for ten and fifteen minute access times). Where populations (in terms of census enumeration districts) are within more than one isochrone they allocated them to the nearest hospital by distance so that all enumeration districts were associated exclusively with one hospital; the most accessible. The 'exclusive' population of a hospital is the population within its ten minute isochrone.

Section 4:   The principles on which this review is based

Contents of this section

4.1: The views of patients and their parents

We agreed at the outset that the views of children, parents and voluntary organisations would be taken fully into account in arriving at our recommendations. We obtained these views in a number of ways:

- **From The welfare of children and young people in hospital.** This report from the Department of Health collates and sets out the principles and standards for the welfare of children in hospital that have been developed over more than 30 years by a wide spectrum of professional and non-professional bodies, including groups like Action for Sick Children (formerly the National Association for the Welfare of Children in Hospital), which represent the views of consumers. This document also formed the basis of our views on quality of service issues.

- **From Children first,** a report from the Audit Commission. This report collates the views of a large number of parents and families on the pattern and quality of health services for children. (We also drew on unpublished material to which we were given access.)

- **From written evidence and telephone calls.** We received a great deal of valuable first-hand information from parents and families about their experiences or perceptions of hospital services, and their views on how things might be improved.

- **From meetings with voluntary organisations and parents' groups.** Members of the Review Group outlined the approach they would be adopting in this review at a series of meetings with interested parties. The sharing of ideas at this early stage was much appreciated by everyone concerned.

The overview that follows was compiled from all the above sources.

Access to services

In general, parents said that the quality of service and the outcome of treatment were their primary concerns, and that access to services was a secondary consideration — indeed, where inpatient admission was required for congenital heart disease or cancer, for example, the accessibility of the service was felt to be a minor consideration.

Many parents said that the location of the major inpatient services in London was relatively unimportant, so long as it was possible for them to stay with (or close by) their child, preferably in accommodation provided by the hospital. However, their support for the principle of fewer but larger treatment centres was qualified. It was clear, for example, that the costs of travelling for treatment or to visit a child in hospital puts an enormous financial strain on many families; fewer centres would exacerbate this problem since some families would have to travel even further. There were also the practical transport difficulties to take into account, especially for those families without a car, and some parents said that being away from home for longer periods would make it harder to arrange for their other young children to be looked after in their absence. It was pointed out that a combination of these factors might prevent some children from getting to a major treatment centre at all.

In the light of these comments, we took the view that **any "package" of care negotiated between a purchaser and a secondary or tertiary level provider should address the possibility of either providing transport or paying the travelling expenses for a child and one escort, both for treatment and visits, and for other appropriate members of the child's family or friends.**

Patterns of care

It is clear that children and parents in the main prefer to deal with staff with whom they have built up a relationship; consequently, treatment at a distant, unfamiliar hospital can be unduly stressful. Parents proposed alternative patterns of care to overcome this problem; outreach clinics, where the parent and child attend at their local hospital, were a popular option. However, it was felt that outreach clinics would only work successfully if parents and children were able to transfer their trust in the major centres to their local services. (Parents of children suffering from serious conditions frequently learn a great deal about their child's condition and worry that local services will not be able to provide the same standards of treatment and care as services provided in a major centre.)

Children and their parents need to be confident that shared management arrangements between the tertiary and secondary levels and the primary and community levels of the service are carefully planned, and that everyone involved has the appropriate skills and knowledge to care properly for the child. Tertiary centres must help to develop the skills of local staff and convey to parents that they can trust their local services.

Standards of care

Some parents were concerned that nationally-recognised standards of care for children might not be met in single-specialty hospitals where paediatric input was minimal. (It was also pointed out that not all secondary level services for children in London meet nationally-agreed standards of care at present.)

Representatives of several consumer groups expressed the view that the development of a full range of child health services at primary and secondary levels should be the overriding aim of all local providers, and that any aspirations to take on tertiary services should be subordinate to this.

Communication and decision-making

Many parents said the frequent breakdowns in communication between the different levels of the health service left them angry, confused and unsure of where to turn for advice. Others said they were concerned about the lack of visual and written information designed specifically for children.

In our view, the sharing of information between professionals and parents can be the first step in establishing a true partnership between them. Parents need sufficient opportunity and information to make informed choices about their child's care; and children, who frequently admit to feeling excluded from decisions about what happens to them, need support and information too.

It needs to be more widely recognised at tertiary, secondary and primary levels that parents and children have a crucial part to play in making decisions about their care.

The needs of adolescents and young adults

The needs of adolescents in hospital are very different from the needs of young children or adults. Many parents said they felt the transfer to adult care was often abrupt and badly managed. It was pointed out that few London hospitals make separate provision for adolescents, even though the Department of Health recommends that separate facilities should be provided for them within paediatric units.

Attitudes to change

Parents and consumer groups were unanimous in their view that services for seriously ill children which are working well and delivering high quality care should not be moved. They expressed a wide range of concerns about the process of managing change, and the consequences of failure for the quality of care. They were particularly concerned about how uncertainty among staff — uncertainty about their jobs and the future of their units — might translate into uncertainty for the children, and how the same uncertainties might affect outside bodies and their investment decisions.

There was a general concern that established teams should not be broken up and have their development work inhibited. The received opinion was that if services **had** to be transferred, then planning should start early, the whole team should be involved, and the full range of services they required (including research and development services) should be provided in their new location.

A major fear — exacerbated by the very tight timetable of the review itself — was that decisions about the future would be made hastily and in an *ad hoc* fashion, resulting in services being "shoe-horned" into inappropriate locations simply to meet arbitrary deadlines.

It was widely recognised that a perfectly viable tertiary service might be undermined by changes in other departments in a hospital and that to prevent this happening planners should take a "holistic" look at the hospital as a whole. The same point held true for hospitals that would be receiving additional services as a result of the adult specialty reviews.

4.2:   The views of health care professionals

Reports published over the last four years reflect a widespread consensus about the standards of care that should be provided for children when they fall ill. We have drawn freely on the principles set out in these reports and have used them as the basis of our own recommendations. We paid particular attention to the Department of Health's guidelines in **The welfare of children and young people in hospital** and the British Paediatric Association's **Towards a combined child health service.**[3] Our debt to the Audit Commission's **Children first** has already been mentioned. Another fundamental source was **Bridging the gaps,**[4] a study of the interfaces between primary and specialist care for children, which was produced on behalf of the influential Caring for Children in the Health Service group.[*]

What follows is a summary of principles from these reports on which we based our recommendations.

---

[*] The parent organisations of the Caring for Children in the Health Service group are the Royal College of Nursing of the United Kingdom, the British Paediatric Association, the National Association of Health Authorities and Trusts, and Action for Sick Children.

A total service

An integrated child health service is concerned with the prevention of illness as well as its cure and involves many different parts of the NHS. In an integrated child health service it is important that:

- the role of each party is clear to the parents of children who use the service, as well as to the staff who provide the service.
- services are provided in a co-ordinated and consistent way.
- wasteful duplication and the inefficient use of resources is avoided.

In the view of the Department of Health, the Welsh Office and many professional bodies, these guiding principles should underpin all child health services.

The different levels of care

Hospital-based and community-based child health services are interdependent. General practitioners and primary care teams provide health care for all children in the context of the family and the home for 24 hours a day. Consultants supported by teams of professionals in the hospital and the community complement the primary care service by providing secondary care for children in the context of the family, the home, school and hospital.

The quality of care

All our sources agreed that a high quality child health service should be based on the following fundamental principles:

- Children have different needs from adults.
- Children are part of a family.
- Children are dependent on their parents for physical and emotional care and support.

It follows that a full range of child health services should provide for the child as a whole, for his or her complete physical and emotional well-being, and not simply for the condition for which treatment or care is immediately required.

The organisation and delivery of care

When a child is transferred into or out of hospital, the following principles should apply:

- Parents should be encouraged to participate in the care of their child.

- Professionals should be prepared to share information so that parents — and children, when they are able — are in a position to make choices and decisions about care.

- Parents should be quite clear about the care they are expected to provide, the point at which they should seek help, and where they can get medical, nursing or other clinical advice and support when they need it.

Printed information should be available for parents and children at every stage: to prepare them in advance of a hospital visit, to keep them informed during it, and to take home with them afterwards. The hospital's "philosophy of care" should be displayed prominently and should be included in the information given to parents.

The full range of child health services

A hospital providing a full range of child health services will have:

- a neonatal service for the surveillance of well babies and therapeutic services, including resuscitation, for new-born babies. (There should be short-term neonatal intensive care in all hospitals and longer-term intensive care in some hospitals.)

- an accident and emergency department with separate admission space for children.

- children's medical and surgical inpatient, day patient and outpatient services, including sessions at peripheral clinics.

- arrangements for paediatric intensive care.

- a full range of children's support services, including therapists, play specialists and teachers.

- arrangements for collaborating with primary care and community health care staff.

- arrangements for collaborating with outside agencies that support families caring for children at home.

- a home nursing service.

The hospital environment for children and their families

Children should be cared for in dedicated areas, not in areas shared with adults. The layout of these areas should take account of the fact that each child is likely to be accompanied by at least one parent. Play space should be provided for young children and recreational areas for older children.

Where facilities have to be shared with adults (for example, in x-ray or imaging departments) there should be staff on hand who are trained in the care of children. The comforting presence of parents in such circumstances can greatly reduce the stress on the child.

Accommodation for parents

Since the majority of parents will choose to stay overnight with their child if given the option, hospitals should make arrangements to accommodate between two-thirds to three-quarters of parents. Three types of accommodation should be available: parents should be able to sleep next to their child's bed, or within sight of it; within "dressing-gown distance" of their child's bed; or away from the ward, if they wish. All such accommodation should be provided free of charge.

The staffing of child health services

Section 6 of **The welfare of children and young people in hospital** offers the following advice on staffing levels:

- Every child admitted to a hospital children's department should be supervised by a children's physician or surgeon. Where, exceptionally, a child has to be admitted to an adult department, a named paediatric consultant should be responsible for advising on the care and treatment of the child.*

---

* The principle that a named paediatric consultant should be responsible for general oversight and advising on the care of children in hospital is entirely supported. However, we acknowledge reservations expressed regarding the advice given in the welfare of children in hospital guidance regarding the assumption of clinical responsibility by a paediatric consultant for all children. At the current time consultant paediatricians would not accept that they are responsible for clinical treatment by surgical specialities.

- There should be at least two registered sick children's nurses — or two nurses who have completed the child "branch" of a Project 2000 education and training programme — on duty 24 hours a day in all children's wards and departments.

- There should be a registered sick children's nurse — or a Project 2000-trained nurse — available 24 hours a day to advise on the nursing of children in the intensive care unit, the accident and emergency department, and outpatients.

- All professional staff who treat or care for sick children should be specifically trained to do so, especially if they usually treat or care for adults, and should know how to communicate sympathetically with parents.

4.3:   The siting of tertiary services

After giving full consideration to the views of parents, patients and professionals, we concluded that **tertiary services for children should be based only in hospitals that can provide a full range of child health services.** This would

- **ensure** that the ethos of the hospital is one which provides for the child as a whole — for his or her complete physical and emotional well-being — and not simply for the condition for which treatment or care is required.

- **ensure** that qualified paediatric staff are readily available to oversee services provided by specialists who normally treat and care for adults.

- **reinforce** the principle of co-ordination between tertiary services and secondary and primary level services.

In view of the financial pressures being exerted on purchasers in London resulting from changes in the system of capitation funding, we consider it unlikely that the cost of meeting the above standards could be justified **unless the hospital in question was serving a sufficient catchment area to generate a significant volume of general paediatric medical admissions.**

We further consider that wasteful duplication and the potentially inefficient use of resources can best be avoided by secondary and tertiary level services sharing access to paediatric intensive care units. (Access to paediatric intensive care units is required by hospitals that provide substantial accident and emergency services, by paediatric surgeons, cardiothoracic surgeons, neurosurgeons, paediatric oncologists, nephrologists, plastic surgeons, and a wide range of other paediatric specialists, such as immunologists and those who deal with infectious diseases.)

4.4: Suggested models of tertiary care

Our terms of reference require us to advise on models of tertiary care; however, since the services we are dealing with are all different, we felt it would be inappropriate to do so. Instead, we outline below the principles that we believe should govern the links between tertiary centres and the populations they serve — the importance of which we have emphasised throughout this report.

In our view a tertiary centre should offer highly specialised care for children with very rare or complex conditions. Such a centre should be based at a hospital where a full range of skills, knowledge, and equipment can be drawn together with associated specialties. However, the services provided by the centre must reach out to the whole population.

The involvement of a tertiary centre in the care of a child will depend upon the child, the type and the severity of the medical condition, the development of sequelae and complications, and the side effects of treatment. In other words, the extent and the nature of the involvement may vary widely and should be managed in different ways at different times. The centre's overall responsibility is to transfer the child back to secondary level care or on to the adult services.

Achieving a balanced service

The mechanism for dealing with the dynamics of tertiary level services should be the contracting process between purchasers (including fund-holding general practitioners) and providers at the primary/secondary and secondary/tertiary level interfaces. Secondary level contracts should include arrangements for tertiary referrals. It is at this stage that the pattern of tertiary services can be shaped with sensitivity to the needs of the local population.

Contracts should aim to produce a balanced service. This might be achieved by providing outreach clinics run by staff from the tertiary centre; by supporting local primary and secondary care professionals; by shared management protocols; or by staff rotation through the tertiary centre.

The most appropriate form of care for rarer conditions might be home support provided by a liaison nurse from the tertiary centre (as often happens now). In such cases the liaison nurse should make sure that the existing primary and secondary care workers are fully involved.

The key to achieving a balanced service lies in the development of shared protocols. Contractual obligations should specify the criteria for the different levels of the service, the availability of resources, staff skills and other aspects of quality of care.

The importance of local contacts

Children with conditions normally requiring treatment at a tertiary centre may occasionally experience less serious problems that can be managed satisfactorily in their local hospital. In such cases the tertiary centre should strive to ensure that patients and their parents retain confidence in their local services by offering them information and advice, and by communicating with their usual professional carers.

The importance of working with a child's school or the local social services should not be underestimated; contacts with these and other agencies may profoundly influence the child's subsequent development, and are all factors in optimising outcome.

4.5: Summary

Taking full account of all the advice received from reports, parents, professionals, consumer groups and voluntary agencies, we reached the following conclusions about the siting of tertiary services in London. These conclusions form the basis for our proposed changes to the pattern of service set out in section 6 of this report.

1. A hospital that aims to provide tertiary services for children should first establish a full range of child health services for the local population.

2. Tertiary services should not be moved to a hospital until that hospital is able to provide a full range of child health services for the local population.

3. Tertiary services should be centred in a hospital, but should reach out to the whole population they serve.

4. Access to tertiary services is a minor consideration when inpatient admission is required during the course of treatment. Most families are primarily concerned with the quality of the service and the outcome of the treatment.

5. The mechanism for dealing with the dynamics of a tertiary service should be the contracting process between purchasers and providers at the primary/secondary and secondary/tertiary level interfaces.

6. The outreach services provided by a tertiary centre should be based on a purchasing strategy that reflects the health needs of local children, rather than on history, tradition or personal contact. In this way tertiary centres will be able to support primary and secondary services in influencing the health of deprived populations in their vicinity.

7. Tertiary centres should develop shared management arrangements to help with the "transfer of trust" from major centres to local services.

8. Relocating services in London will require the highest level of skill. Parents fear that failure to manage change properly will result in a loss in the quality of care for their children.

References

1. Department of Health, **The welfare of children and young people in hospital,** London, 1991
2. Audit Commission, **Children first,** London, 1993
3. British Paediatric Association, **Towards a combined child health service,** London, 1991
4. Rosemary Thornes, **Bridging the gaps,** Caring for Children in the Health Service (Consortium Report) London, 1993

Section 5:   The specialty reviews

Contents of this section

5.1: Children's cancer services (paediatric oncology)

The specialty

Children's cancer services provide care for children with tumours arising in solid tissues in any part of the body and also management of blood cancers such as leukaemia.

Estimates of need

The expected number of children aged 0-14 years with cancer in each of the four Thames regions (estimated from national rates) is 269 a year — see Table 3 at the end of this section. This figure is slightly lower than the 290 cases a year given in the report of the United Kingdom Children's Cancer Study Group. The difference may be due to several factors. It could be

- because the calculation of case numbers is not based on age-specific rates.
- because the incidence of cancer is higher in the 0-5 years age group.
- because the percentage of children under five years of age is now higher than it was in the 1970s (the latest period for which aggregate data has been analysed).

Based on these figures, we believe that treatment will be required for 250-300 children each year.

The trend over the past 20 years has been increasingly to centralise care for children with cancer into regional paediatric oncology centres. This trend has not been universal, however, and it has been possible to study the differences in survival rates for children who have been referred to a major centre and those who have not.

The Childhood Cancer Research Group has shown that there is a significant improvement for many cancers when care is centralised. There are some cancers (Wilms' s tumour, for example) for which the benefits of centralised care cannot be demonstrated; even so, patients with these cancers are still better off being treated by a major centre. There is evidence to show that patients who are not referred to a major centre are often treated with out-dated therapies which "over-treat" them, thus causing unnecessary and unwanted late effects.

Because childhood cancer is a rare disease, no single cancer centre in the UK is large enough to conduct random studies on its own patients. Instead, different centres collaborate on large co-operative studies, and the majority of children in the UK are entered into therapeutic studies run by either the Medical Research Council or the United Kingdom Children's Cancer Study Group. Again, there is evidence from the Childhood Cancer Research Group to show that children entered into such studies have a better chance of survival and of receiving the most appropriate and up-to-date therapy.

The overall cure rate for childhood cancer is now over 60%; for some cancers, such as acute lymphocytic leukaemia, it is over 90%. Successful treatment can bring its own problems, however, and long-term follow-up studies have shown that many children suffer from renal and cardiovascular dysfunction, problems with fertility, secondary tumours, neuropsychological sequelae, and social problems, including difficulties with schooling.

Advice received from paediatric oncologists

The United Kingdom Children's Cancer Study Group recommends:

- Children with cancer should be referred to a major centre that can offer specialist skills in the treatment of both the cancer and the child.

- The minimum number of new patients for a specialist service should be 50-60 a year.

- Each major centre should have facilities for the intensive treatment of the cancer at tertiary level. Facilities for less intensive therapy should be provided in district general hospitals on a shared management basis with appropriate support services.

- Specially-trained children's nurses should provide outreach care and family support.

- There should be easy access to the ancillary disciplines of social work, physiotherapy, pharmacy, dietetics and nutrition.

The UKCCSG advises that paediatric ICU, radiology haematology, pathology, and nephrology should be on-site and that essential linkages should be established with radiotherapy, cardiology, gastroenterology endocrinology, ENT/audiology, adult haematology but that these services can be off-site. It is not essential to have links with adult oncology.

In a joint report, four paediatric oncologists (one from each United Kingdom Children's Cancer Study Group centre) have suggested that two or three major cancer centres with a minimum of two full-time paediatric oncologists in each would be an appropriate level of service for London.

Current provision

There are currently four United Kingdom Children's Cancer Study Group centres in London. These are at:

- St Bartholomew's Hospital.
- Great Ormond Street Hospital.
- The Royal Marsden Hospital (Sutton).
- University College/Middlesex Hospital.

To some extent the four centres complement each other:

- St Bartholomew's Hospital provides a national service for children with retinoblastoma.
- Great Ormond Street Hospital has a particular interest in leukaemia and lymphoma. Bone marrow transplants are carried out here.
- The Royal Marsden Hospital has developed high-dose chemotherapy. Bone marrow transplants are carried out here.
- University College/Middlesex Hospital provides a service for adolescents with brain and bone tumours.

According to NHS regional data, children with cancer (including leukaemia) are also treated in other hospitals in the four Thames regions — at district general hospitals like Northwick Park Hospital and Hillingdon Hospital, for example, and at teaching hospitals such as the Royal Free Hospital and the Royal London Hospital. Some of the children treated in these hospitals may be part of shared care arrangements. In addition, a significant number of children with brain tumours are seen in the neurosurgical units at Atkinson Morley's Hospital, at Charing Cross Hospital, and at Guy's Hospital. Bone marrow transplants are carried out at the Royal Free Hospital, the Hammersmith Hospital, St George's Hospital and the Royal London Hospital. Some children with liver cancer are managed at King's College Hospital.

Of all the children with cancer on the United Kingdom Children's Cancer Study Group register who were referred from the four Thames regions in 1990 and 1991, 36% were seen at Great Ormond Street Hospital, 20.9% at the Royal Marsden Hospital, 16.4% at St Bartholomew's Hospital, and 9.6% at University College/Middlesex Hospital — see Table 4 at the end of this section. For a significant number of children from the South West Thames region, the service appears to be provided from Southampton.

Current workload

Data for 1991/92 obtained from the hospitals' own administration systems was based on numbers of completed consultant episodes rather than individual cases. We decided it would be preferable to rely on the data on the number of new cases from the provider units themselves, even though we had no means of cross-checking its accuracy. The data for oncology is summarised in Table 5 at the end of this section and includes referrals from outside the four Thames regions.

At present, Great Ormond Street Hospital is the largest centre and treats the largest number of patients; the Royal Marsden Hospital is the second largest centre but has a significantly smaller workload; St Bartholomew's Hospital and the University College/Middlesex Hospital both treat fewer patients than the Royal Marsden Hospital, especially when the highly specialised workloads for retinoblastoma and bone marrow transplant are excluded from the figures.

Conclusions and recommendations

After weighing up all the information about paediatric oncology available to us, we concluded that:

1. All children with cancer should have the benefit of care from a specialist children's cancer service.
2. For the four Thames regions, with a child population of 2.6 million and between 250-300 new patients a year, two tertiary centres would be sufficient but three or four could be justified.
3. The future concentration of services should enhance existing standards, aid teaching and research, and have the advantage of economy of scale.

On the basis of these conclusions, we recommend that tertiary level inpatient services for children with cancer in London should be concentrated in two or three tertiary centres.

Our suggestions about where these centres should be located are given in section 6.

5.2:   Children's cardiology and cardiothoracic services (paediatric cardiology)

The specialty

Paediatric cardiac services care for new-born babies and children with diseases of the heart and circulation, both congenital and acquired. This includes outpatient and inpatient admission, non-invasive and invasive investigation, and all necessary surgical services.

Estimates of need

Seven or eight babies in every thousand suffer from congenital heart disease. About half of these require surgical treatment at some time, and many operations are performed during the first year of life. This proportion is likely to increase in parallel with advances in medical and surgical management.

In recent years there has been some reduction in complex cardiac disease in early infancy as a result of antenatal diagnosis and termination of pregnancy. This has led to a reduction in waiting list figures, but probably not to a decrease in workload yet. There has been no reduction in the number of children requiring surgery for congenital heart disease. (This may reflect the increasing expertise and type of operations available for this age group.)

The UK surgical register records a national rate of about 70 open and closed heart operations on children per million population each year, which is equivalent to about 1,000 surgical procedures in the four Thames regions each year.

The outlook for most children needing cardiac surgery is now so good that they may well have a fairly normal life-span and quality of life. This has led to a need for cardiologists who are able to provide long-term care for adolescents and young adults with congenital heart disease.

A small number of patients do not stand to benefit from advances in conventional surgery and their outlook is poor. For these patients heart transplantation has recently become a possibility.

Advice received from paediatric cardiologists

Paediatric cardiologists consulted by the Review Group made the following recommendations:

- Children with diseases of the heart and circulation should be treated only in hospitals with a full range of child health services.

- Paediatric cardiologists should have ready access to a comprehensive range of specialist and sub-specialist services, notably adult cardiology, fetal medicine and neonatal medicine. Genetics, cardiothoracic surgery, nephrology, paediatric intensive care and neuroscience should also be available.

- Provision should be made for interventional catheterisation techniques and electrophysiological investigation and treatment, including ablation therapy.

○   The concentration of medical expertise and resources should be sufficient to maintain clinical expertise and provide teaching and research opportunities, yet should avoid the duplication of expensive services.

○   Peripheral outreach clinics from the paediatric cardiology centre are an essential part of any service.

○   Diagnostic and treatment units for fetal cardiology should be an integral part of all paediatric cardiology services.

The British Paediatric Cardiology Association recommends a minimum of one consultant paediatric cardiologist per million population. This equates to four cardiologists in each cardiac centre in the south-east of England. The Association further recommends that two cardiothoracic centres should serve London and the south-east.

Current provision

Paediatric cardiac services are currently offered at four hospitals in London:

- Great Ormond Street Hospital.
- Guy's Hospital.
- Harefield Hospital.
- The Royal Brompton Hospital.

The services offered at each hospital are as follows:

- Great Ormond Street Hospital has a full range of cardiothoracic services and is one of only three children's heart transplant units in the UK. It is developing fetal cardiology services and ECMO*, and provides a number of outreach cardiology clinics. There is capacity for a further 300 cardiac operations each year.

- Guy's Hospital has a full range of cardiothoracic services and a well-developed fetal cardiology service, including neonatal and paediatric intensive care. There are close links with the adult cardiothoracic service and there is on-site support from paediatric renal and neurology services. It also provides outreach cardiology clinics. There is spare inpatient capacity.

---

* ECMO (Extra Corporeal Membrane Oxygenator) - a high technology treatment for babies with severe respiratory problems.

- Harefield Hospital offers paediatric cardiology, cardiac surgery — with considerable expertise in transplantation — and an intensive care unit. It has no other services for children.

- The Royal Brompton Hospital has a full range of cardiothoracic services (including ECMO) housed in a new building with a paediatric respiratory unit and a paediatric cardiac intensive care unit, but no other paediatric services. It also provides a number of outreach cardiology clinics. There are close links with the adult cardiothoracic and respiratory services. The new Chelsea and Westminster Hospital, which offers a wide range of paediatric specialties, is situated close by. The Royal Brompton Hospital has the capacity to perform 60% more cardiac operations a year.

Current workload

Data obtained from the hospitals and the regional information services was based on numbers of completed consultant episodes rather than individual cases. This data was of variable quality and limited value (one hospital did not even distinguish between investigations and operative procedures). The paediatric cardiology workload is shown in Table 6 at the end of this section. We also received information on the number of open and closed heart operations and this is also shown at Table 6. From the returns submitted by each hospital we calculate that the patients were referred from the following sources.

Great Ormond Street Hospital	**Total from Thames regions = 51%**
Guy's Hospital	**Total from Thames regions = 88%**
Royal Brompton Hospital	**Total from Thames regions = 80%**

Conclusions and recommendations

After weighing up all the information about paediatric cardiology available to us, we concluded that:

1. Paediatric cardiology and cardiothoracic services in the Thames regions can be accommodated in two centres.

2. There is spare capacity in London.

3. Harefield Hospital is a single specialty hospital which is isolated geographically and offers no other paediatric services.

On the basis of these conclusions, we recommend that inpatient cardiology and cardiothoracic services at tertiary level in London should be concentrated in two or possibly three tertiary centres.

Our suggestions about where these centres should be located are given in section 6.

5.3: Paediatric neurology and neurosurgery

The specialty

Paediatric neurology comprises acute paediatric neurology and work with chronic neurological disability, both of which form a regional service. Acute paediatric neurology involves management of children, for example, with acute encephalopathy. Work with chronic neurological disability includes work with rare neurodegenerative disease, complex and rare neuro developmental problems and neuromuscular disease.

Paediatric neurosurgery meets two main needs, for children with neural tube defects, brain tumours, cranio-facial defects and epilepsy, and for children with head injury. Paediatric neurosurgery should be based in a specialist centre providing comprehensive services for children, and provided by surgeons with special training in paediatric neurosurgery.

Essential links are with neuro-radiology, neuro-physiology and paediatric neuro-anaesthesia. Paediatric intensive care is essential for the management of major head injuries and also following elective operations for brain tumours or epilepsy. Links with plastic surgery are necessary for cranio-facial surgery and with A&E for trauma.

Estimate of need

It was not possible to distinguish clearly between the need for paediatric neurology at secondary and tertiary levels so no assessment could be made on a population basis. Some children with rare, complex or degenerative disorders need care from a specialist tertiary centre.

At least one third of all children in intensive care units have neurological problems, and 5-10% suffer from neurological disorders following cardiac surgery (the figure is higher when new techniques such as ECMO are being developed).

Advice received from paediatric neurologists

The British Paediatric Neurology Association believes acute paediatric neurology should be a regional service. Work with children with chronic neurological disability is part of a regional service, but the majority of such children should be managed locally with support from the regional paediatric neurology centre when necessary. The Association made the following recommendations:

- Paediatric neurology services should be provided only in hospitals with a full range of child health services.

- A paediatric neurosciences centre should combine neurosurgery with tertiary paediatric neurology and supporting paediatric neurophysiology and neuroradiology and paediatric anaesthesia and intensive care. Specialist biochemistry, neuropsychiatry, neuropathology and neuro-ophthalmology are important components of the service.

- Paediatric neurologists should have ready access to intensive care and to radiotherapy, orthopaedic, ophthalmology, audiology, psychiatry and clinical genetics services. Paediatric paramedical and nursing support is essential.

- There should be other tertiary services for children on the same site, including oncology, infectious diseases, growth and endocrinology services, and cardiology.

The British Paediatric Neurology Association recommends a minimum of three whole-time equivalent consultant paediatric neurologists to serve a regional population of three to four million.

Current provision

There are currently two major centres within the four Thames regions providing a comprehensive paediatric neurology service. These are at:

- Great Ormond Street Hospital
- Guy's Hospital

Paediatric neurologists work in isolation at St George's Hospital, St Mary's Hospital and the Chelsea and Westminster Hospital, and there is a neuromuscular service at the Hammersmith Hospital. Other hospitals providing services for children with disability include the Royal London Hospital and King's College Hospital; these have not been included in this review as they appear to be largely district-based services. (The Royal Free Hospital identified a paediatric neurology workload but is not listed by the British Paediatric Neurology Association as a paediatric neurology centre.)

At present paediatric neurosurgery is provided in 10-12 hospitals. All of them, apart from Great Ormond Street, are adult units. These are listed in Table 7 at the end of this section.

Current workload

Data obtained from the hospitals' own patients administrative systems for 1991/92 was based on numbers of completed consultant episodes rather than individual cases. For children's neurosurgery the data from regional sources seemed more secure and has been used instead. The table below gives some idea of the workload:

Unit	New Out Patient	Old Out Patient	IP FCE	Comment
Great Ormond St	600	2,000	1,000	
Guy's			828	special out patient figures
Chelsea & Westminster	190	400	120	
St George's	280	330	100	
Hammersmith	total =	1500	200	

The hospitals supplied the following additional information:

- Great Ormond Street Hospital has 900-1,000 neurosurgical admissions each year, of which only 1.5% are from acute head injuries.

- Atkinson Morley's Hospital had 217 paediatric neurosurgical admissions in 1991/92. About 28% were for head injuries.

- The Maudsley Hospital had 132 admissions for neurosurgical procedure on children in 1991/92, of which 12% were following trauma. Children are transferred to Guy's Hospital for post-operative intensive care.

Conclusions and recommendations

After weighing up all the information about paediatric neurology and neurosurgery available to us, we concluded that:

1. Neuroscience centres should be based only in hospitals with a full range of child health services.

2. Neurosurgery should be carried out only in such centres.

3. Children with a head injury must be admitted to a hospital providing comprehensive services for children. There must be firm links to a paediatric neurosurgical service; children with head injury who require intensive care, with or without an operation, should be referred to a specialist paediatric centre providing paediatric intensive care and neurosurgery.

On the basis of these conclusions, we recommend that tertiary paediatric neurology and neurosurgery services should be concentrated in two or possibly three tertiary level neuroscience centres serving London and the Thames regions.

Our suggestions about where these centres should be located are given in section 6.

5.4 Nephrology (renal medicine)

The specialty

Renal services for children include acute and diagnostic nephrology, the management of end-stage renal failure and paediatric urology. The association between congenital disorders of the urinary tract and mal-development or damage to the renal parenchyma leads to a greater dependency between paediatric nephrology and urology than in adult practice and these services might be regarded as different aspects of the same discipline. Paediatric nephrology centres should provide renal transplantation and chronic dialysis.

Estimates of need

Estimates of the number of children with end-stage renal failure requiring treatment by kidney transplantation in the UK are quoted in the 1979 report by the British Association for Paediatric Nephrology. This cites an incidence of 1.3-3.5 children aged 0-15 years per million of the population - or 7-10 patients per million children, which is in the order of 100 new patients a year.

The Association's latest report estimates that approximately 3 children aged 0-15 years per million of the total population with end-stage renal failure which is approximately 42 children a year in the four Thames Regions.

Advice received from paediatric nephrologists

The paediatric nephrologists we consulted advised that:

- Paediatric nephrology centres should be distributed so that all children have access to expert care.

- Paediatric nephrology centres should have a catchment area sufficiently large to maintain clinical expertise.

- Peripheral clinics held jointly with paediatricians at district general hospitals are essential to reduce travelling times for parents and children.

- Specialist children's renal nurses are essential in each designated centre. Each centre should also have access to all necessary support services (registered children's nurses, social workers, dietitians, psychologists, psychiatrists, teachers, play therapists, etc)*

- Haemodialysis should be carried out in an independent children's dialysis unit adjacent to a children's ward or in a children's hospital. Peritoneal dialysis and training for home treatment should be carried out on the children's ward or in the children's dialysis are carried out should have access to paediatric high dependency and intensive care.

There are clinical and academic advantages for both the adult and paediatric nephrology services to be located on the same site, but this is not a pre-requisite for the paediatric nephrology service; where this is not the practice, close contact should be maintained through joint meetings and audit (this will make it easier to transfer patients from paediatric to adult services). Close collaboration with paediatric urologists is, however, essential in the management of surgical conditions that threaten the upper renal tract. Management of neuropathic bladder should be shared by the paediatric nephrologist and the urologist.

Current provision

There are currently three paediatric nephrology centres in London. These are at:

- Great Ormond Street Hospital
- Guy's Hospital
- The Royal Free Hospital

The services offered at each hospital are as follows:

- Great Ormond Street Hospital provides a comprehensive service for children of all ages presenting with any variety of nephro-urological disease or related disorders. It has a chronic dialysis and transplant programme for children, and its outreach services include a home CAPD (Continuous Ambulatory Peritoneal Dialysis) programme and regional specialty clinics. Twenty-three per cent of the hospital's workload in this specialty comes from outside the four Thames regions, notably from Oxford region and East Anglia region (neither of which has its own paediatric nephrology service).

---

* A multi-disciplinary approach is necessary in view of the problems of growth failure, delayed puberty, non-compliance and psychosocial maladjustment in the presence of chronic disease.

Important note: The nephrology units at Great Ormond Street Hospital and the Royal Free Hospital (see below) are regarded as a joint department. Children under 5 years of age in end-stage renal failure are managed at Great Ormond Street Hospital; those over 5 years old are managed at the Royal Free Hospital. The urology department at Great Ormond Street Hospital also functions as one unit with the urology service at the University College/Middlesex Hospital (which treats older children and adolescents and has close links with adult urology and renal programmes).

- Guy's Hospital provides a regional paediatric nephrology and urology service for the South East Thames region and a large part of the South West Thames region. It also provides renal transplantation and all forms of chronic dialysis for children with chronic renal failure in the South East Thames, South West Thames and Wessex regions.

- The Royal Free Hospital has four cubicles equipped for haemodialysis, a day care area and a school adjacent to the general paediatric ward, which is shared by children with renal problems. (The paediatric nursing staff who care for children with renal problems also attend children with haematology disorders.) After having a transplant, children are nursed in a discreet area in the post-operative ward and usually return to the children's ward in 48 hours. In the adult dialysis unit there is a separate area for children's haemodialysis. The hospital provides outreach paediatric nephrology clinics in both the North East Thames and North West Thames regions.

Current workload

Data obtained from the regional information service was based on numbers of completed consultant episodes rather than individual cases. This data was of limited and variable quality; we judged it preferable to rely more on the data sent directly from the provider units themselves, although we had no means of cross-checking its accuracy. The table below shows the inpatient and outpatient activity and the number of transplants each year:

Unit	In patient	Out patient	Transplant pa
Great Ormond Street	1077	2902	8
Royal Free	282	1663	13
Guy's	1170	2300	15-40

Conclusions and recommendations

After weighing up all the information about paediatric nephrology available to us, we recommend that there be two centres for paediatric nephrology in London and the Thames regions with the continuation of an extensive outreach service supporting children nearer their homes.

5.5   Plastic Surgery and Burns

The Specialty

Paediatric plastic surgery (and where relevant, maxillo-facial and oral surgery) consists of specialist surgery for children with congenital abnormalities and general plastic surgery. Cleft palate and cranio facial malformations for example, require specialist plastic surgery and trauma and minor congenital abnormalities, for example, require general plastic surgery.

Estimates of need

We have undertaken no estimates of need for this specialty.

Advice Received

Paediatric plastic surgery must be provided by surgeons with special training in the specialty based in a hospital providing a full range of services for children. Specialist surgery should be provided in a specialist children's centre.

Paediatric burns units require 4-6 beds for a population of 5 million, linked to specialist children's services, including paediatric intensive care. Most children with burns are treated as outpatients and appropriate facilities dedicated to children are necessary.

Essential links are with paediatric anaesthesia and for specialist plastic surgery with paediatric intensive care and the full range of children's services. There should be links with paediatric neurosurgery for cranial-facial surgery and with A&E for trauma.

Current provision and workload

The four centres for plastic surgery undertake the highest volume of plastic surgery for children as follows:

Hospital	Finished Consultant Episodes For Children 1991/92
St Andrew's (Billericay)	1,065
Queen Victoria (East Grinstead)	797
Queen Mary's (Roehampton)	832
Mount Vernon	702

The other hospitals undertaking more than twenty Finished Consultant Episodes (FCEs) on children in 1991/92 were:

Hospital	Finished Consultant Episodes 1991/91	Comments
Great Ormond St/ Queen Elizabeth (Hackney)	510	Cleft palate repair Cranio facial service (this is supra-regional service)
University College/ Great Ormond Street	106	Including adolescents from Middlesex
Royal London	91	Including cleft palate and hand surgery
Guy's/St Thomas'	436	Including cleft palate and hand surgery
King's College	34	
St George's	152	
Charing Cross	237	Including cranio-facial surgery

Children with burns are treated at St Andrew's, Queen Victoria, Guy's and University College/Middlesex.

Conclusions and recommendations

We recommend that:

1.   Specialist plastic surgery should be consolidated onto two or three sites. These would include Great Ormond Street and Guy's/St Thomas'.

2.   General plastic surgery for children should be undertaken in hospitals with a full range of child health services available.

We have not as a group considered the location or size of burns units in London. On the basis of advice received and stated above two paediatric burns units, each with six to eight special care paediatric beds and outpatient services based on hospitals with a full range of child health services, would appear to meet the needs of the population of the Thames regions.

5.6   Neonatal and specialist paediatric surgery

The specialty

The specialty covers neonatal surgery, specialist paediatric surgery, paediatric general surgery and paediatric neurology.

Neonatal surgery is required for the surgical treatment of infants of 44 weeks conceptual age or less.

Specialist paediatric surgery is required for major surgery in children. Examples include re-section of tumours, hepato-biliary surgery, operations for major gastro-intestinal abnormalities and reconstructive surgery following operations performed in the neo-natal period.

Paediatric general surgery is the surgical treatment of children with conditions such as congenital inguinal hernia, hydrocele, circumcision, undescended testis, umbilical hernia, pyloric stenosis, appendicitis, testicular torsion, incarcerated inguinal hernia.

Paediatric urology is a sub-specialty within specialist paediatric surgery.

Estimates of need

We have undertaken no estimates of need in this specialty.

Advice received

The British Association of Paediatric Surgeons recommends one paediatric surgeon per 500,000 total population and the King's Fund one per 750,000. On this basis the Thames regions would require between twenty and twenty-eight paediatric surgeons. Urological conditions of childhood should be treated by trained paediatric urologists.

In addition to the full range of child health services the hospital on which the paediatric service is based must provide paediatric anaesthesia, paediatric intensive care, dedicated operating theatres and paediatric radiology.

There should be strong links with easy access to gastroenterology, nephrology, neurosciences, cardiology, oncology, plastic surgery, ear, nose and throat and orthopaedic surgery.

For neonatal surgery there must be a neonatal intensive care unit in addition to these facilities and links with pre-natal and genetics services. The critical mass for a neonatal surgical service is one hundred major neonatal operations annually, supported by two intensive care cots.

General paediatric surgery may be provided outside a paediatric surgical centre in a hospital with general paediatric services. Essential requirements are a general surgeon and an anaesthetist with special training in paediatric surgery, paediatricians, a paediatric ward and an intensive care unit with facilities for children. The caseload must be adequate to maintain expertise.

Current provision and workload

North central sector

Neonatal surgery is currently offered at:

- Great Ormond Street which has a nine cot surgical neonatal intensive care unit and operated on 142 major cases in 1991/92.

- University College which treats about 25 major cases a year and has a neonatal intensive care unit.

Paediatric surgery is currently offered at:

- Great Ormond Street which operated on 1,136 paediatric surgical and 1,111 paediatric urological patients in 1991/92 more than 90% of these being specialist paediatric surgical patients.

- University College/Middlesex which provides a specialist paediatric surgical service for urology and oncology in the field of both brain and bone tumours.

North east sector

Neonatal surgery is currently offered at:

- Queen Elizabeth Hospital which undertook 108 major cases in 1991/92 and has a surgical neonatal intensive care unit.

Paediatric surgery is currently offered at:

- Queen Elizabeth Hospital which undertook about 1,600 paediatric surgical procedures in 1991/92 and was supported by a surgical paediatric intensive care unit.

- Royal London Hospital which provides some specialist services provided by adult surgeons in the field of neurology, ear, nose and throat and plastic surgery.

- St Bartholomew's offers limited specialist services provided by adult surgeons in support of specialist paediatric services in the fields of gastroenterology and oncology.

South east sector

Neonatal surgery is currently offered at:

- Guy's with approximately 30 non-cardiac neonatal surgical cases per annum with a neonatal intensive care unit.

- King's College Hospital with about 30 major cases annually plus 30 neonatal liver operations - supported by a neonatal unit.

- Lewisham with 87 major cases in 1991/92 supported by a neonatal intensive care unit

- St Thomas' with less than 20 operations a year with a neonatal intensive care unit.

Paediatric surgery is currently offered at:

- Guy's/St Thomas' - in 1992 the two units had 766 paediatric surgical FCEs.

- King's - the emphasis is on the complex hepato-biliary surgery with some specialist and general paediatric surgery. It currently has 2 PICU beds expanding to 4 in August 1993 (these are currently supported by two high dependency beds expanding to 4 by August).

- Lewisham - paediatric surgical and urological activity was 994 FCEs in 1991/92.

Brighton has 2 paediatric surgeons providing specialist paediatric and neonatal surgery.

South west sector

Neonatal surgery is currently offered at:

- St George's Hospital had 120 major cases in 1992 supported by a neonatal intensive unit.

Paediatric surgery is currently offered at:

- St George's which provides the inpatient paediatric surgical service supported by a three bedded paediatric intensive care unit. Day care surgery is also undertaken. This service has recently been transferred from Queen Mary's Carshalton.

North west sector

Neonatal surgery is currently offered at:

- Chelsea and Westminster Hospital with 38 neonatal and a further 68 patients aged 1-3 months reported.

- Hammersmith Hospital which performed an estimated 30 neonatal operations annually.

Paediatric surgery is currently offered at:

- Chelsea and Westminster with 948 FCEs now supported by two paediatric intensive care beds situated in the adult intensive care unit.

- Hammersmith with approximately 350 FCEs in 1991/92.

- St Mary's with approximately 400 paediatric surgical procedures performed annually.

Conclusions and recommendations

We have concluded that paediatric surgical services in London have developed haphazardly over five decades.

In 1987 the King's Fund report on paediatric surgery in Greater London identified thirteen paediatric surgeons working at thirteen hospitals and made recommendations for rationalising paediatric surgical services in London. Despite this, in 1993 there are fifteen paediatric surgeons providing services at twelve hospitals. With the establishment of new neonatal surgical services outside London the number of referrals to London hospitals is decreasing.

In some hospitals the number of both neonatal surgical and paediatric surgical cases treated are small and the consultant sessional cover in some sectors is fragmented.

We do not believe the current fragmentation is conducive to high quality of service nor to the effective use of specialist surgical, anaesthetic and nursing resources. The lack of concentration of paediatric intensive care beds has difficulties in coping with fluctuations in demand and maintaining team work.

We recommend that:

- One paediatric surgical centre should be established in each of the five sectors.

- This centre should be based at a hospital providing a full range of child health services and the essential requirements for both paediatric surgery and neonatal surgery.

- Specialist paediatric surgery and neonatal surgery should be consolidated in the paediatric surgical centre for each sector.

5.7   Paediatric Intensive Care

Overview

A paediatric intensive care unit provides for the treatment and management of children from four weeks of age to adolescence, regardless of the specialty involved. Although most sick neonates are managed in neonatal intensive care units and in special care baby units, there are some with special requirements - such as those who have had major surgery - who may be cared for in a paediatric intensive care unit.

The Paediatric Intensive Care Society advises that paediatric intensive care should be provided on a regional basis, and that general paediatric intensive care units will usually be additional to the paediatric sub-specialty units for cardiothoracic surgery and neurosurgery.

The Society recommends a minimum of one general paediatric intensive care bed per 40,000 of the child population (but this may be an underestimate). A paediatric intensive care unit should have at least four beds and admit a minimum of 150 patients a year.

A paediatric intensive care unit must have:

- Facilities for artificial ventilation, invasive cardiovascular monitoring, renal support, intra-cranial pressure monitoring and complex intravenous nutrition and drug scheduling;

- immediate access to all radiological and imaging facilities, including ultrasound and CT scanning;

- ready access to expert microbiological, biochemical and haematological advice. All necessary blood products must be available;

- a staff which includes paediatricians, paediatric anaesthetists and registered children's nurses, all trained in paediatric intensive care;

- a fully equipped transport team for the safe retrieval and transfer of critically ill infants and children to and from other hospitals.

ANALYSIS OF DISTRIBUTION OF PAEDIATRIC SPECIALTIES IN LONDON HOSPITALS

Specialty	King's	St George's	Chelsea & Westminster	Royal London	Queen Elizabeth	St Mary's	University College/Middlesex	St Bartholomew's	Guy's & St Thomas'	Royal Free	Hammersmith	Charing Cross	Great Ormond Street	Royal Brompton
Cardiology	✓								✓				✓	✓
Neurosurgery		✓AMH										✓	✓	
Renal									✓	✓			✓	
Neurology	✓	✓	✓	✓?					✓		Muscle		✓	
Cardiac Surgery									✓				✓	✓
Endocrinology	✓						✓	✓					✓	
Gastroenterology			✓		✓			✓	✓				✓	
Infectious Diseases		✓			✓	✓	✓						✓	
Immunology	✓	✓			✓	✓	✓		✓				✓	
Haematology	✓	✓			✓		✓		✓	✓	✓		✓	
Oncology					✓		✓	✓	✓				✓	
Paediatric Intensive Care	✓	✓	✓		✓	✓			✓				✓	✓
Respiratory	✓				✓				✓		✓		✓	✓
Metabolics		✓	✓	?✓			✓		✓				✓	
Rheumatology		✓	✓						✓				✓	
Paediatric Surgery	✓	✓	✓		✓	✓			✓		✓		✓	

Specialist Plastic Surgery: Queen Mary's
Mount Vernon
Queen Victoria
St Andrews

Burns: Billericay
East Grinstead
Guy's
University College/Middlesex

Current provision

The preliminary results of a national survey carried out by the British Paediatric Association Working Party on Paediatric Intensive Care suggests that paediatric intensive care is provided in eleven hospitals in inner London:

- Chelsea and Westminster Hospital
- Great Ormond Street Hospital
- Guy's Hospital
- King's College Hospital
- Lewisham Children's Hospital
- Queen Elizabeth Hospital, Hackney
- Queen Mary's Hospital, Carshalton
- Royal Brompton Hospital
- Royal London Hospital
- St George's Hospital
- St Mary's Hospital

King's College Hospital, the Queen Elizabeth Hospital, Hackney and the Royal Brompton Hospital have paediatric intensive care units in support of liver surgery, paediatric surgery and cardiothoracic specialty work, respectively.

Recommendations

Each PICU should have at least four beds and be accepting a workload of in excess of 150 children a year. The population of London would justify the provision of five paediatric intensive care units. The requirements of the other specialty services for paediatric intensive care are in addition to these numbers.

Those units providing cardiac and neurosurgery for children should be located with general paediatric intensive care units in a tertiary care comprehensive centre.

5.8   Other specialist services

We have concentrated on the tertiary services listed in sections 5.1 to 5.7. There are a range of other specialist services for children and details of their location are shown on the opposite page. For these services we have included an overview and a statement on the current provision in the this section. We have made no recommendations on their future disposition but indications of their linkages with other specialties can be obtained by cross referencing.

Endocrinology

Overview

Endocrinology services are required to meet the considerable demands from growth surveillance and assessment and from those who provide c are for children with diabetes. Services are also needed to deal with genital anomalies, complicated growth disorders, pituitary deficiency, adrenal and thyroid disorders, and oncology/endocrine disorders.

Endocrinologists need links with oncologists, regional screening programmes, metabolic services, neurosurgeons, surgeons, gynaecologists and urologists.

The British Society for Paediatric Endocrinology recommends that there should be at least one and preferably two paediatric endocrinologists in each region.

Current provision

Paediatric endocrinology services are currently provided at three hospitals in London:

- St Bartholomew's Hospital
- Great Ormond Street Hospital
- University College/Middlesex

Great Ormond Street Hospital and the University College/Middlesex Hospital are hoping to develop a centre for paediatric endocrinology, and there is a 'loose federation' being formed between the paediatric endocrinologists at the University College/Middlesex Hospital and St Bartholomew's Hospital. King's College Hospital and the Chelsea and Westminster Hospital receive endocrine services from the University College/Middlesex Hospital. St George's Hospital is developing its own paediatric endocrinology service. At the Royal London Hospital, one consultant paediatrician provides a district based endocrinology service with an adult endocrine specialist. Guy's Hospital provides its own service. There is an extensive network of outreach clinics.

Gastroenterology

Overview

The British Society of Paediatric Gastroenterology and Nutrition recommends that each region should have at least one identified referral centre for children with gastrointestinal, liver and nutritional disorders, and that this should be provided in a children's unit. Regional centres should provide liver biopsy, isotope scanning, pancreatic function testing and specialised biochemistry testing;

a dedicated paediatric endoscopy unit and a day care unit are also highly desirable. The Society advises that children should be admitted to the regional

centre for intensive investigation but management thereafter in outreach clinics by paediatricians based at their local district general hospital.

Gastroenterologists need links with paediatric surgeons, radiologists, clinical chemists, child psychiatrists, histopathologists and immunologists, all of whom should be on the same site. Expert dietetic advice is essential for nutritional support.

The British Society of Paediatric Gastroenterology and Nutrition recommends that there should be three major hepatology centres in the UK and that each region should have two consultants to provide adequate cross-cover.

Current provision

Tertiary level gastroenterology services are provided at:

- St Bartholomew's Hospital
- Chelsea and Westminster Hospital
- Great Ormond Street Hospital
- King's College Hospital
- St George's Hospital

St Bartholomew's Hospital is a leading centre for research in paediatric gastroenterology (closely linked with adult gastroenterology); it has a particular interest in inflammatory bowel disease, as does the Queen Elizabeth Hospital, Hackney. Great Ormond Street Hospital has a particular interest in mobility and King's College Hospital has a supra-regional liver unit. St Thomas' Hospital provides a service for constipation and bowel mobility problems.

The pattern of referrals to these hospitals take account of the type of patient problems rather than regional boundaries.

Metabolic disease

Overview

Because metabolic disorders are rare, the British Society of Paediatric Gastroenterology and Nutrition says it is likely that two or three centres will be sufficient to meet the needs of the UK. These should be located in a tertiary level centre providing a full range of child health services, including specialist laboratory and dietetic support services.

The paediatric specialities necessary for the care of children with metabolic and liver disease include ophthalmology, cardiology, infectious diseases, immunology, nephrology and gastroenterology. Paediatricians with a special interest in metabolic disease have an important role in the identification of those children needing referral.

Current provision

Great Ormond Street is regarded as the national centre for the investigation of complex metabolic disease. It is supported by specialist laboratories at Guy's Hospital, the University College/Middlesex Hospital, Charing Cross Hospital, St George's Hospital and the Institute of Child Health. At Great Ormond Street there are close links between the department of clinical biochemistry, the paediatric intensive care unit and the department of neurology for metabolic neurological disorders. There are consultants with a special interest in metabolic disease at St George's Hospital, Guy's Hospital and the Chelsea and Westminster Hospital.

Haematology

Overview

Although the vast majority of common haematological conditions are managed at district level by haematologists and paediatricians, we were advised that there is a requirement for tertiary level centres with diagnostic and treatment facilities for children with rare congenital bone marrow disorders, aplastic anaemia, leukaemia, lymphoma and myelodisplasia, including bone marrow transplantation, and for children with disorders of coagulation and haemoglobin synthesis. We were also advised that a close relationship between paediatric oncology and haematology is essential, and that high quality district services are required for children with haemoglobin disorders, particularly where there are high concentrations of patients from ethnic minorities.

Current provision

At present bone marrow transplants are carried out at Great Ormond Street Hospital, the Hammersmith Hospital, the Royal London Hospital, the Royal Marsden Hospital, the Royal Free Hospital and St George's Hospital (St George's has a special interest in bone marrow failure syndromes).

Great Ormond Street Hospital has a multi-disciplinary paediatric haemophilia unit; the Royal London Hospital, the Royal Free Hospital and St Thomas' Hospital also have haemophilia units, but these are not multi-disciplinary. The Royal Free has recently appointed a paediatric haematologist for children with haemophilia.

There are sickle cell and thalassaemia clinics at King's College Hospital, the University College/Middlesex Hospital, Queen Elizabeth Hospital, Hackney, and the Central Middlesex Hospital

Paediatric rheumatology

Overview

Northwick Park Hospital is the only London Hospital specialising in paediatric rheumatology; it is considered a national resource. There is great interest in rheumatological disorders at Great Ormond Street Hospital and St George's Hospital has a paediatric rheumatology clinic. District general hospitals where an adult rheumatologist holds a joint clinic with a paediatrician include Lewisham Hospital, the Royal London Hospital, Queen Elizabeth Hospital, Hackney and Chase Farm Hospital.

Infectious diseases

Overview

The British Paediatric Association recommends that children with severe or unusual infections or infectious diseases should be managed by paediatricians with an expert understanding of host/microbial interaction. It also advises that policies for the control and prevention of infections, especially those related to immunisation and AIDS, should be determined by paediatric infectious diseases specialists, and that clinical immunologists should be closely involved in the care of children with immuno deficiency diseases. Paediatric infectious diseases specialists need access to paediatric and neonatal intensive care, haematology, immunology, neurology and paediatric surgery.

The British Paediatric Association recommends a minimum of two consultant paediatricians in paediatric infectious disease per region.

Current provision

There are currently three hospitals in London with children's infectious diseases unit:

- Great Ormond Street
- St George's Hospital
- St Mary's Hospital

In addition, Queen Elizabeth Hospital, Hackney, provides a service linked to its department of gastroenterology, while University College/Middlesex Hospital is interested in children who suffer from sexually transmitted diseases, including HIV.

Respiratory medicine

Overview

The British Paediatric Respiratory Group recommends that each region should have one respiratory medicine centre to deal with acute respiratory problems, chronic complex respiratory diseases (including asthma), congenital lung abnormalities, cystic fibrosis, sleep studies and post-intensive care management of acute lung disease. The centre should have respiratory laboratories capable of providing a complete range of measurement services for all ages, including infant lung function, skin tests, exercise testing and comprehensive sleep studies. The centre should support cardiothoracic units where heart and lung transplants are carried out.

Current provision

There are currently five hospitals in London providing services in respiratory medicine:

- Great Ormond Street Hospital
- Guy's Hospital/St Thomas' Hospital
- Hammersmith Hospital
- King's College Hospital
- Royal Brompton Hospital

The Queen Elizabeth Hospital, Hackney, and Great Ormond Street Hospital refer children with cystic fibrosis to King's College Hospital and the Royal Brompton Hospital. The Children's Hospital, Lewisham also provides a service.

Orthopaedic surgery

Paediatric orthopaedic surgery consists of specialist surgery in fields like scoliosis, neuro-muscular disorders associated with cerebral palsy, abnormal gait and bone tumours and general surgery including trauma. It should be provided by surgeons with special training in paediatric orthopaedics and based in hospitals with a full range of child health services.

Essential links with paediatric anaesthesia and paediatric intensive care for bone tumours must be linked with a paediatric oncology centre.

Current provision

Specialist paediatric orthopaedic services are provided by:

- Great Ormond Street
- University College/Middlesex
- Royal London
- Guy's/St Thomas'
- Royal National Orthopaedic Hospital, Stanmore

Each of these hospitals have particular interests.

Ear, nose and throat surgery

Overview

Specialist ENT surgery includes surgery of the larynx, tanchea and inner ear and the management of neonatal airway obstruction.

ENT surgery should be provided by surgeons with special training in ENT surgery based at a hospital with a full range of child health services. Essential links are with paediatric (ENT) anaesthesia and for specialist ENT surgery with paediatric intensive care and other specialist paediatric services.

Current provision

Specialist ENT surgery is provided at:

- Great Ormond Street
- Guy's/St Thomas'

Ophthalmology

Overview

Paediatric ophthalmology is a tertiary specialist service which includes the management of retinopathy of prematurity, tumours, congenital glaucoma and cataract and strabismus. Surgeons managing children should have special training in paediatric ophthalmology and provide their services in a hospital with a full range of child health services. Essential links are with ophthalmology support services eg optics and with paediatric anaesthesia and neurology.

Current provision

Specialist ophthalmology services are provided at:

- Great Ormond Street
- Moorfields

TABLE 3

REFERRAL PATTERNS IN THE THAMES REGIONS

TO UKCCSG CENTRES

1990-1991

**Expected Number of Cases of Cancer in 1991 in
Children aged 0-14 years
Thames Regions Only**

Four Thames Regions	M * O - 14	1,340,858	153	= 269
	F * O - 14	1,273,100	116	
North West Thames	M * O - 14	340,458	39	= 68
	F * O - 14	323,310	29	
North East Thames	M * O - 14	374,200	43	= 75
	F * O - 14	355,200	32	
South East Thames	M * O - 14	350,700	40	= 70
	F * O - 14	334,200	30	
South West Thames	M * O - 14	275,500	31	= 55
	F * O - 14	260,400	4	

TABLE 4

CHILDREN WITH CANCER ON THE UKCCSG REGISTER

REFERRED FROM THE FOUR THAMES REGIONS

IN 1990 AND 1991

(TWO YEARS)

Centre	NEW	NWT	SET	SWT	Total
St Bartholomew's	37	21	32	5	95
Great Ormond Street	69	48	77	18	212
Royal Marsden (Sutton)	0	9	23	90	122
University College Middlesex	17	21	6	6	50
Other UKCCSG Centres*	4	10	2	4	20
Other Hospitals	23	21	18	20	581
TOTALS	150	130	158	143	581

*   eg Cambridge and Southampton

Source: Charles Stiller, Childhood Cancer Research Group, Oxford

TABLE 5

PAEDIATRIC ONCOLOGY: DATA FROM PROVIDER UNITS

1991/92 (ONE YEAR)

Hospital	New Cases per annum	Source
Great Ormond Street	130	Most from 4 Thames RHAs
Royal Marsden (Sutton)	120	Majority from SWTRHA
St Bartholomew's	100	35% have retinoblastoma
University College Middesex	71	Could include GOS transfers

TABLE 6

PAEDIATRIC CARDIOLOGY WORKLOAD

Returns from each Unit

(twelve months workload)

Unit	Intervention	Open	Closed	TOTAL
Great Ormond Street	104	450	260	814
Guy's	98	141	48	287
Royal Brompton	150	370	370	520

OPEN AND CLOSED HEART OPERATIONS

1991 - THAMES DISTRICT HEALTH AUTHORITIES

Hospital	Number of Open Heart Operations	Number of Closed Heart Operations	Total
Great Ormond Street/Hospital for Sick Children	417	143	560
RBH	309	85	394
Harefield	169	42	112
Guy's	112	43	155

NEUROSURGERY FROM REGIONS 91/92

DATA age 0-14

Admissions as coded

TABLE 7

PROVIDER	ALL	HEAD INJ (HI)	% HI	CRANIOTOMY CODES	TUMOUR CODES	IC OPS NOT HI	IC OPS HI
Charing Cross	76	49	35.5	48	16	61	6
Thames RES Rx Outside	52	33	36.5	13	7	18	4
SBH	28	22	21.4	13	18	10	3
Oldchurch	30	13	56.7	13	0	3	7
Middlesex	11	11	0	0	14	2	0
Brighton	1	1	0	15	2	15	0
All Saints	0	0		0	9	0	0
Brook	4	0	100	2	1	0	2
SGH	221	162	26.7	54	9	38	18
Mid Sussex Hos	14	9	35.7	4	0	6	3
QMH Children	0	0		9	5	10	0
QMH ROE	0	0		0	21	1	0
RLH	60	39	35	18	11	13	9
RLH	19	16	15.8	7	0	9	3
RFH	44	26	40.9	12	1	7	4
GOS	695	682	1.9	94	148	0	0

Section 6: A review of current services and proposals for change

Contents of this section

6.1: The service providers by sector

In this section we review the services currently available in inner London and identify the actions which, in our view, are necessary to create the full range of child health services upon which tertiary centres should be based.

For the purposes of this review we have divided inner London into five sectors, as follows:

Sector	Teaching hospital	Special health authority	District general hospital
North Central	The Royal Free Hospital	Hospital for Sick Children, Great Ormond Street	Whittington Hospital
	University College/ Middlesex Hospital	National Hospital for Nervous Diseases	
North East	St Bartholomew's Hospital		
	Homerton Hospital The Royal London Hospital	Queen Elizabeth Hospital, Hackney	
South East	Guy's Hospital/ St Thomas's Hospital	The Bethlem and Maudsley Hospital	Lewisham Hospital
	King's College Hospital		
South West	Atkinson Morley's Hospital	The Royal Marsden Hospital (Sutton)	St Helier Hospital
	St George's Hospital		Queen Mary's Hospital, Carshalton
North West	Charing Cross Hospital	The Hammersmith Hospital	
		The Royal Brompton Hospital	
	The Chelsea and Westminster Hospital	The Royal Marsden Hospital	
	St Mary's Hospital		

6.2: North Central Sector

The district health authority in this sector is the purchasing authority for people living in the London Borough of Camden and the London Borough of Islington. With a total resident population of 348,000, this sector is the most densely populated per hectare in inner London. It has a child population of 69,000 (19.9%).

The hospitals relevant to us in this sector are:

- The Hospital for Sick Children, Great Ormond Street.
- University College/Middlesex Hospital.
- The Royal Free Hospital.
- The Whittington Hospital.

The Tomlinson report estimated the "exclusive population" of the University College/Middlesex Hospital as 80,153 adults and children, and of the Royal Free Hospital as 144,186 adults and children.

The Hospital for Sick Children, Great Ormond Street*

Profile

Great Ormond Street Hospital provides a complete range of tertiary services for children and is the largest single provider in the four Thames regions of all the main tertiary services covered in this review. It has particular expertise in caring for very young children. (Some of the other tertiary centres told us that they always referred their very young patients to Great Ormond Street Hospital.) It also provides a range of supra-regional services and undertakes around 14,000 episodes of inpatient care a year. Further detail is given in Appendix 2.

Commentary

In our view Great Ormond Street Hospital is a regional, national and international asset that should be developed further. Internationally, it projects an image of caring and clinical excellence for the NHS and the country as a whole. It earns income by providing services for children from countries which are not able to establish specialist services for themselves. Furthermore, the volume of work undertaken at Great Ormond Street Hospital and the associated Institute of Child Health make it a suitable site for research and development work, and one with the potential to accommodate the variations in workload associated with research.

---

* The Hospital for Sick Children, Great Ormond Street, is commonly referred to simply as "Great Ormond Street Hospital". In order to avoid confusion, we have adopted this title throughout this report.

Great Ormond Street also makes a very significant national contribution to the training of children's nurses.

However, Great Ormond Street Hospital does not have an accident and emergency department or a GP admissions unit; it does not have a maternity unit or neonatal medical service; and it does not have sufficient services for adolescents. Nor are there any fully developed links with specialist services for adults.

Accidents are a major health problem for all children, and head injuries are a significant cause of death and disability; indeed, over 95% of children who are admitted to hospital under the care of paediatricians are presented as emergencies. If Great Ormond Street Hospital is to be a centre of excellence it must be able to address the challenging problems that such admissions create.

Furthermore, many of the conditions that require expert major surgery in infancy can now be recognised before birth, and pre-birth diagnosis is likely to improve this even further. Since the management of many surgical problems now begins before birth, close proximity to a maternity service or tertiary surgical service will become increasingly important.

A hospital also needs to be able to meet the requirements of children as they grow — both in size and in their need for independence — or to have appropriate arrangements for them with another unit.

In the light of these considerations, we concluded that Great Ormond Street Hospital should provide secondary level child health services to its local population. One way of doing this would be to introduce GP admissions or an accident and emergency service. However, opening an accident and emergency service would probably result in the hospital being flooded with children from all over London, so we discounted this option. (We understand the hospital is now accepting a limited number of GP referrals.)

In **Making London better**, the Government expressed its wish to see further progress towards a greater integration of services between the University College/Middlesex Hospital, Great Ormond Street Hospital and the National Hospital for Neurology and Neurosurgery. This would begin to correct some of the deficiencies of Great Ormond Street Hospital as well as building on the strengths of the University College/Middlesex Hospital. (We were advised, however, that the number of accident and emergency attendances to the University College/Middlesex Hospital is only 60,000 a year, and that the proportion of children is only around 11% of this number.) In our view, the arrangements for secondary level services provided for local residents by the Royal Free Hospital and the Whittington Hospital should also be reviewed. The following options should be considered:

Option 1: to concentrate children's inpatient facilities on two sites — Great Ormond Street Hospital and the Whittington Hospital.

Option 2: for Great Ormond Street Hospital to staff the children's wards that back up the accident and emergency departments at the University College/Middlesex Hospital, the Royal Free Hospital and/or the Whittington Hospital.

Option 3: for Great Ormond Street Hospital to concentrate on children below, say, 10 years of age, and the University College/Middlesex Hospital or the Royal Free Hospital to concentrate on adolescents.

Option 4: to concentrate neonatal intensive care on one site to which Great Ormond Street Hospital is linked.

We do not underestimate the implications of these options for the hospitals concerned. Great Ormond Street Hospital has little experience in the secondary level market[*], whereas the Royal Free Hospital has one of the lowest costs for paediatric medical admissions in London.

We further recommend that:

1. The neuromuscular service is transferred from the Hammersmith Hospital to Great Ormond Street Hospital.

2. The specialist rheumatology service is transferred from Northwick Park Hospital to Great Ormond Street Hospital.

3. The retinoblastoma service is transferred from St Bartholomew's Hospital to Great Ormond Street Hospital.

These are all national services that fit into Great Ormond Street Hospital's national role. (In the light of the discussions we had with parents and voluntary organisations, we would suggest that it takes care to ensure that the facilities required by these three services can be accommodated properly, and this will take time.) We believe the hospital should give priority to developing the links we have suggested for secondary level services.

---

[*] Though it did indicate to us that it felt it could be competitive in the tertiary care market providing its excess costs were reimbursed within 5% of the level assessed.

Summary

We believe our recommendations will improve services for the local population and maintain and develop services at Great Ormond Street Hospital. From the point of view of children's services, changes to the management arrangements between the University College/Middlesex Hospital and Great Ormond Street Hospital may improve the chances of integration. We recommend that Great Ormond Street Hospital should remain a major centre for children's cardiothoracic services, cancer services, neurosciences, nephrology and plastic surgery services (the latter to be established in conjunction with an adult department).

We also confirm our general view that all these services should be provided on the basis of contracts that serve specific populations, and that appropriate models of care should be developed for them.

University College/Middlesex Hospital

Profile

There are 27 children's beds at University College Hospital and 15 at the Middlesex Hospital. The University College/Middlesex Hospital has an accident and emergency department, a maternity service, a neonatal unit, an intensive care unit and a fetal medicine unit. Tertiary services for children are provided in endocrinology, immunology, haematology, oncology, metabolic, neurology and plastic surgery and burns. Children with brain tumours are referred to the radiotherapy unit by neurosurgeons at Great Ormond Street Hospital. The hospital also provides a special service for children with bone tumours. Further detail is given in Appendix 2.

Commentary

In our view the general hospital services for children at the University College/Middlesex Hospital are too small to support a full range of child health services. It has been suggested that the University College/Middlesex Hospital might unite with the Royal Free Hospital; should this happen, some rationalisation of existing services could take place in conjunction with our proposals for links with Great Ormond Street Hospital.

We recommend that:

1.   University College/Middlesex Hospital should link its paediatric services with those at Great Ormond Street Hospital.

2.   University College/Middlesex Hospital should concentrate on providing a quality outpatient or day care service. This could be provided without inpatient responsibilities, or at a level required to support the accident and emergency service only.

3.   Children who require immediate admission or longer-stay care should be transferred from the University College/Middlesex Hospital to Great Ormond Street Hospital. The wards that accommodate these children at present should be adapted to take only older children; all children below a certain age should go to Great Ormond Street Hospital.

We believe the links between the University College/Middlesex Hospital and Great Ormond Street Hospital could be enhanced by changes in the management arrangements, and in particular by the appointment of a single clinical director for the two hospitals.

Summary

We have recommended that there should be a single clinical director providing the neonatal service at the University College/Middlesex Hospital, that secondary level and other services should be provided at Great Ormond Street Hospital, that there should be a back-up ward to support the accident and emergency department, and that tertiary services for adolescents should be provided in conjunction with the Royal Free Hospital. If these recommendations are implemented, we believe the following advantages would accrue:

- There would be an improvement in the quality of service for local children.

- University College/Middlesex Hospital would have access to the full support facilities of Great Ormond Street Hospital.

- Children requiring paediatric surgery would no longer have to be transferred from the University College/Middlesex Hospital to Queen Elizabeth Hospital, Hackney.

- The University College/Middlesex Hospital medical school would have a sound base for undergraduate teaching.

- Postgraduate teaching would benefit from unique access to expertise in infant, child, adolescent and adult medical care.

The Royal Free Hospital

Profile

The Royal Free Hospital has 30 children's beds, a maternity unit and a neonatal intensive care unit. It has developed a community-oriented child health service and provides a tertiary service in paediatric nephrology, renal surgery, haemophilia and haematology. It has the second largest renal transplant service in the UK, and children over two years of age are transferred here from Great Ormond Street Hospital for transplants. It has outreach clinics in east and north Hertfordshire and in north-east London. Further detail is given in Appendix 2.

Commentary

The Royal Free Hospital provides a relatively small general paediatric service. We have recommended elsewhere in this report that nephrology and renal surgery should be concentrated in two centres, one of which should be at Great Ormond Street Hospital. Any inpatient paediatric haematology should be accommodated elsewhere.

We recommend that the Royal Free Hospital should link its paediatric services with those at Great Ormond Street Hospital and concentrate on providing a quality outpatient and community service, either without inpatient responsibilities, or at a level required to support the accident and emergency service only.

Summary

We suggest that the Royal Free Hospital should provide tertiary facilities for adolescents, depending on which tertiary services are placed there following the reviews of adult specialist services.

We further suggest that consideration should be given to linking the management arrangements for children's services at the Royal Free Hospital with the University College/Middlesex Hospital and Great Ormond Street Hospital.

The Whittington Hospital

Profile

The Whittington Hospital is located geographically in the area covered by the former Islington Health Authority, though the people who use it live mainly in neighbouring Haringey. It provides a general paediatric medical service and a maternity service, and it has a neonatal intensive care unit. It has no other tertiary services. Further detail is given in Appendix 2.

Commentary

The Whittington Hospital is relevant to this review only inasmuch as it is a major service provider at secondary level. As such, its views will have to be considered fully if our recommendations for links between the University College/Middlesex Hospital, the Royal Free Hospital and Great Ormond Street Hospital are implemented. The Whittington Hospital is likely to be a "key player" in any changes instigated by local purchasers seeking to ensure that there is a full range of child health services for the local population.

6.3:   North East Sector

The district health authority in this sector is the purchasing authority for people living in the City of London, the London Borough of Hackney, the London Borough of Newham and the London Borough of Tower Hamlets. The total resident population of this sector is 569,400. It has a child population of 135,650 (23.8%).

The hospitals in this sector are:

- St Bartholomew's Hospital.
- The Homerton Hospital.
- Newham Hospital.
- Queen Elizabeth Hospital, Hackney.
- The Royal London Hospital.

The Tomlinson report estimated the "exclusive population" of St Bartholomew's Hospital as 34,775 adults and children, and of the Royal London Hospital as 139,070 adults and children.

The proportion of children in the population in this sector is the highest in inner London, and the level of social deprivation (as measured by the Townsend scores) is also very high. Work carried out in the West Midlands has shown that at these levels of deprivation there is a risk that children will not have the access to hospital care that they require. In our view the overriding priority of purchasers and providers in the North East Sector should be to develop a full range of child health services for the local population and to integrate these services at primary and secondary levels.

Within this framework we are recommending that the Queen Elizabeth Hospital, Hackney, should be moved on to the same site as the Royal London Hospital as a matter of urgency (see below) to create one local hospital with a full range of child health services at secondary care level.

St Bartholomew's Hospital

Profile

St Bartholomew's Hospital has a 22-bed children's ward. It provides a small-scale general paediatric service but no maternity services. Its strength lies in its provision of three tertiary level services for children — oncology, gastroenterology and endocrinology. It is one of the four cancer treatment centres recognised by the United Kingdom Children's Cancer Study Group in south-east England, and it is a national centre for the treatment of eye tumours (retinoblastoma).

In the past a substantial number of children have been transferred from Great Ormond Street Hospital to St Bartholomew's Hospital for radiotherapy, but there are now plans to transfer this work to the University College/Middlesex Hospital. The number of new paediatric oncology cases treated at St Bartholomew's Hospital is between 80-100 a year, of which 35 are retinoblastomas. Further detail is given in Appendix 2.

Commentary

St Bartholomew's Hospital does not at present provide a full range of child health services and does not serve a population of sufficient size to support such a range. Its emphasis is on teaching and research but it does not have expertise in a number of disciplines associated with children's services; nor does it have a children's intensive care unit.

Those who currently provide the service told us they wished to stay where they were; while the parents of children who use the service were concerned about change, particularly about breaking up excellent teams.

We accept that to move tertiary services would be disruptive — but we do not believe it is inevitable that their quality would fall; indeed, it is possible that the quality might improve.

Summary

We recommend that:

1. The retinoblastoma service should be transferred from St Bartholomew's Hospital to Great Ormond Street Hospital. This is a national service that would fit in well with Great Ormond Street Hospital's national role.

2. The paediatric oncology service should be transferred from St Bartholomew's Hospital to either Guy's Hospital/St Thomas's Hospital, or to St George's Hospital, where it can be linked with services at the Royal Marsden Hospital (Sutton).

3.   Children's services at St Bartholomew's Hospital and the Royal London Hospital should be brought under the management of a single clinical director.

We further suggest that consideration is given to providing outpatient and day care services on the St Bartholomew's Hospital site. This should be provided from the Royal London Hospital.

The Homerton Hospital

Profile

The Homerton Hospital provides a general service to the local population. It has a sizeable maternity unit and a busy neonatal intensive care unit. Children who present at the accident and emergency department are transferred to the Queen Elizabeth Hospital, Hackney, if they require admission as in-patients. There are two consultant neonatologists but no other consultant paediatricians on site. Further detail is given in Appendix 2.

Commentary

Making London better recommended that the management of the Homerton Hospital and the Queen Elizabeth Hospital, Hackney, should be merged to provide a fully-integrated paediatric service for the local population. We understand fully the basis for this recommendation; however, if it were to be acted upon, it is our view that no single hospital in this part of London would be in a position to develop a full range of child health services. We recognise that a paediatric service is required at the Homerton Hospital to support its maternity and neonatal care services to meet the needs of the local population. **Making London better** anticipated that the Royal London Hospital would be linked for service and education to the Homerton and Newham General Hospitals (paragraph 67) and we believe that these should be major links in the case of the Homerton. (See also our comments on the Queen Elizabeth Hospital, Hackney, below.)

Summary

We recommend the establishment of an outpatient and daycare service to meet the needs of the local population in this part of London. We believe that these should be sited at the Homerton Hospital. Wherever sited these services should be served on an outreach basis by the Queen Elizabeth/Royal London Hospitals.

Newham Hospital

Profile

Newham Hospital has 38 children's beds, a large maternity unit and a neonatal intensive care unit. It provides a general medical paediatric service. Further detail is given in Appendix 2.

Commentary

We mention Newham Hospital only for the sake of completeness in this sector.

Queen Elizabeth Hospital, Hackney

Profile

This hospital is a major provider of secondary level children's services in this sector. It offers a general paediatric service, a plastic surgery service, a major paediatric surgical service, and paediatric intensive care as well as tertiary services in gastroenterology, clinical haematology and respiratory medicine (including immunology). Queen Elizabeth also has a paediatric A&E service which provides a major contribution to primary care in this locality. Further detail is given in Appendix 2.

Commentary

We heard good reports of the service provided at the Queen Elizabeth Hospital, Hackney, from local general practitioners. However, the hospital cannot remain where it is indefinitely: it is isolated, serves children only, and the buildings are in a poor state of repair.

Making London better recommended merging the Queen Elizabeth Hospital, Hackney, with the Homerton Hospital in order to provide a fully-integrated paediatric service for this area. Having examined the profile of services provided by Queen Elizabeth Hospital we believe that the needs of local children will best be served by integrating the services at Queen Elizabeth with those at the Royal London. (See also our comments on the Homerton Hospital, above.)

Queen Elizabeth Hospital provides some tertiary as well as secondary services. The transfer to the Royal London rather than the Homerton will allow development of these services together with other tertiary services at the Royal London. A wide range of child health services will then be available to the population served.

Association with adult tertiary services will be close and siting of them within the teaching hospital will advance the opportunities for undergraduate and post-graduate teaching and research. These advantages would not be achieved by relocating Queen Elizabeth Hospital to the Homerton Hospital.

The merged service would have to provide a full paediatric service to the Homerton Hospital; this would have to include outpatient and day care facilities as well as services for well babies and back-up for the accident and emergency department. Since the proportion of children in the population is so high and their needs are so great, it will probably be necessary to re-provide outpatient and day care facilities on — or close to — the Queen Elizabeth Hospital site.

Summary

We recommend **as a matter of priority** that the services currently provided at the Queen Elizabeth Hospital, Hackney, are transferred in their entirety to the Royal London Hospital. This would create a hospital with a full range of child health services at secondary level.

The Royal London Hospital

Profile

The Royal London Hospital has 36 children's beds in a new children's unit (which also contains 10 closed beds). It also provides a maternity service and has one of only two designated neonatal intensive care units in the North East Thames region. The birth-rate is average for a district general hospital, but the paediatric service is small since many local people use the Queen Elizabeth Hospital, Hackney, instead. Further detail is given in Appendix 2.

Commentary

The Royal London Hospital does not at present provide a full range of child health services. Our recommendation to move all the paediatric services currently provided at the Queen Elizabeth Hospital, Hackney, to the Royal London Hospital (see above) would bring together the full range of maternity services and children's services on one site. By adding the paediatric surgical services from Queen Elizabeth Hospital, the Royal London Hospital would become the paediatric surgical centre for this part of London.

The merged service would have to provide a full paediatric service for the Homerton Hospital; this would have to include outpatient and day care facilities and back-up for the accident and emergency department. Outpatient and day care services would also be required on the Queen Elizabeth Hospital site, and possibly also at St Bartholomew's Hospital, subject to local evaluation.

The site development plans for the Royal London Hospital will have to be worked through carefully if children are to receive the maximum benefit from our recommendations. The impressive new unit at the Royal London Hospital will not be large enough to meet all requirements, and proper paediatric intensive care facilities will be needed to support the paediatric surgical service in particular.

Summary

In our view the Royal London Hospital should develop a full range of child health services for the North East Sector of inner London. Having achieved this, it would be in a good position to develop tertiary services for children. The local purchaser should develop the appropriate models of care.

As well as improving the quality of service for local children, we believe our recommendations are in the best interests of undergraduate and postgraduate medical education and will provide a sound foundation for the training and development of doctors and other professional staff.

6.4: South East Sector

The district health authority in this sector is the purchasing authority for the people living in the London Borough of Lambeth, the London Borough of Lewisham and the London Borough of Southwark. The total resident population of this sector is 700,000. It has a child population of 139,000 (19.6%).

The hospitals in this sector are:

- Guy's Hospital/St Thomas' Hospital.
- King's College Hospital.
- Lewisham Hospital.
- The Maudsley Hospital.

The Tomlinson report estimated the "exclusive population" of Guy's Hospital as 75,969 adults and children, of St Thomas's Hospital as 84,373 adults and children, and of King's College Hospital as 265,723 adults and children.

Guy's and St Thomas' Hospital Trust

Profile

We were told that children's services at Guy's Hospital and St Thomas' Hospital would be focused on a single site. At present both sites have their own accident and emergency departments, children's wards, maternity units and neonatal intensive care services and are functioning as separate units. The number of births implies a much larger population base than is evident from the number of paediatric medical admissions; this suggests that women who have their babies in these hospitals go elsewhere for paediatric care.

Guy's Hospital and St Thomas' Hospital have professors and support a staff in paediatric nephrology, paediatric cardiology and cardiac surgery, paediatric neurology and neonatal medicine. Between them the hospitals also provide tertiary services in the fields of gastroenterology, immunology, haematology, respiratory medicine, metabolics, rheumatology, paediatric surgery, plastic surgery, burns and neurology. The paediatric cardiology and nephrology services provide a wide range of outreach clinics, mainly in Kent, Sussex and outer London, and some in East Anglia. Further detail is given in Appendix 2.

Commentary

We were impressed by the determination of those at Guy's Hospital/St Thomas' Hospital to become the second major centre for tertiary services in south-east England. Having said that, we believe their determination needs to be balanced by an equal desire to provide secondary level services for their local population. Objective judgements about service development need to be made by people from outside the Guy's and St Thomas' Hospitals NHS Trust. *

We were also concerned about the combined effects of the site merger and the possible consequences of the adult specialty reviews. We wondered whether the merger (on whichever site is chosen) would work to the patients' advantage, and what effect the changes would have on the environment for patients, relatives and staff.

We recommend that:

> 1. The paediatric nephrology service should remain on the Guy's Hospital/St Thomas' Hospital site.

Thomas's

---

* Although it is not part of our terms of reference, we feel there is a need for a review by the local purchasing authorities in conjunction with the local providers on how a full range of child health services might be provided for the local population in this sector. The aim would be to ensure that service provision was co-ordinated and complementary.

2.   Paediatric neurosurgery should be established on the Guy's Hospital/St Thomas' Hospital site to link up with the existing paediatric neurology services.

3.   The Guy's Hospital/St Thomas' Hospital site should be one of the options for the relocation of the paediatric oncology service from St Bartholomew's Hospital.

4.   The Guy's Hospital/St Thomas' Hospital site should be one of the two options for paediatric cardiology and cardiothoracic services (the other option being the Royal Brompton Hospital, to which the service currently provided at Guy's Hospital could be transferred).

5.   These services will require support from paediatric surgery and the arrangements for this will need to be considered.

Bringing together the children's services of Guy's Hospital and St Thomas' Hospital on one site will produce a strong base for service, education and research at tertiary level. However, our recommendations for the transfer of paediatric oncology and neurosurgical services will put pressure on whichever site is finally chosen, and this will be increased by the recommendations of the adult services review.

Summary

Despite the attractions of locating a full range of tertiary services on one site (which would serve the South East Thames and South West Thames regions and offer competition to Great Ormond Street Hospital), our options for cardiology and cardiothoracic and oncology services should be carefully assessed — as should the overall site plan and costs — before a final decision is made. We suggest a review of child health services is undertaken to determine how best the full range of child health services might be provided locally.

King's College Hospital

Profile

King's College Hospital has a total of 62 children's beds, 18 of which are devoted to hepatology. It has a maternity unit, a neonatal intensive care unit and a

paediatric intensive care unit. The hospital's strengths include hepatology, respiratory medicine and gastroenterology. The hospital has a major interest in sickle cell and haemoglobinopsyhy. There are professors of paediatric hepatology, respiratory medicine and community paediatrics and the head of the department has a major interest in gastroenterology.
Further detail is given in Appendix 2.

Commentary

Deciding between Guy's Hospital, St Thomas' Hospital and King's College Hospital as the primary site for tertiary services in the South East Sector was difficult. We preferred King's College Hospital — it has a full range of child health services with good links to the community and it probably serves as large a local population as any teaching hospital in London — but we found it was not favoured by the adult specialist services review groups.

Summary

We recommend that King's College Hospital builds on its strengths as a district general hospital by developing a full range of child health services. We further suggest that it develops an advanced model of shared care and outreach services by working closely with the tertiary centres.

The Maudsley Hospital

Profile

The Maudsley Hospital provides a neurosurgical service mainly for the South East Thames region. It has an eight-bed children's unit and a rehabilitation unit and specialises in the treatment of epilepsy. Consultant paediatric cover is provided from King's College Hospital. A proposal to develop a neurosciences unit for adults and children linked to King's College Hospital was frozen some years ago. Further detail is given in Appendix 2.

Commentary

We recommend that the neuroscience services currently provided at the Maudsley Hospital are transferred to Guy's Hospital/St Thomas' Hospital to link up with the neurological services there.

Lewisham Hospital

Profile

Lewisham Hospital has 60 children's beds in three wards — paediatric, intensive care and neonatal intensive care. It is a designated paediatric surgery centre for the South East Thames region. Further detail is given in Appendix 2.

Commentary/Summary

Lewisham Hospital provides a full range of child health services for a significant local population. It is also a designated centre for paediatric surgery in South East Thames and serves a much wider population in this area. Since it meets our criteria as a base at which tertiary services can be placed, there is no reason why paediatric surgery should not continue to be based here although detailed arrangements on paediatric surgery input to the tertiary centre and services would need to be worked out if this option is followed.

6.5: South West Sector

The district health authority in this sector is the purchasing authority for people living in part of the London Borough of Wandsworth. The total resident population of this sector is 191,200. It has a child population of 34,000 (17.8%).

The hospitals in this sector are:

- Atkinson Morley's Hospital.
- St George's Hospital.

The South West Sector also includes the Royal Marsden Hospital (Sutton), but this is in outer London in the area covered by Merton and Sutton Health Authority.

The Tomlinson report estimated the "exclusive population" of St George's Hospital as 273,000 adults and children.

Note: The review of acute services set up by South West Thames RHA will as a result of **Making London better** cover resident populations within the boundaries of the Kingston, Richmond, Merton, Sutton and Wandsworth local authorities, and resident populations served by Kingston Hospital, Queen Mary's Hospital, Roehampton, St George's Hospital and St Helier Hospital. We suggest that this review considers how a full range of child health services at secondary level might be provided for these populations.

Atkinson Morley's Hospital

Profile

Atkinson Morley's Hospital has six children's beds. It is a key provider of neurosurgical services for children in south-east England. Further detail is given in Appendix 2.

Commentary

We did not visit Atkinson Morley's Hospital. However, we know from information provided that, as a single-specialty hospital, it does not meet our criteria for a tertiary centre. It is important to ensure that the standards we have outlined are met in respect of the paediatric support for the requirements of children admitted to Atkinson Morley.

In the short term we recommend:

- that St George's Hospital and the host purchaser should review the arrangements for children at Atkinson Morley's Hospital and strengthen the paediatric input, if required.

Elsewhere in this report we recommend that a second neurosciences centre is established on the Guy's Hospital/St Thomas' Hospital site. Assuming that this is established prior to Atkinson Morley's Hospital being moved to another site, we recommend that:

- As soon as a neurosciences centre for children is established at Guy's Hospital/St Thomas' Hospital, children should cease to be admitted to Atkinson Morley's Hospital.

We further recommend that:

- The site to which Atkinson Morley's Hospital is finally relocated should be one with a full range of child health services. So the option of a third neurosciences centre for children can be maintained.

The Royal Marsden Hospital (Sutton)

Profile

The Royal Marsden Hospital (Sutton) provides cancer services for children in the area covered by the Royal Marsden Special Health Authority. It is one of the four

United Kingdom Children's Cancer Study Group centres in south-east England. A new purpose-built children's unit was opened in February 1993. Further detail is given in Appendix 2.

Commentary

The Royal Marsden Hospital (Sutton) provides a high quality cancer service but does not — and cannot — meet our criteria for a tertiary centre. It is our view that services should be moved to a hospital providing a full range of child health services. This may have to be a long term objective as the services are capital intensive and recently provided. Nor does there appear to be alternative spare capacity available.

Summary

Since it would be impractical to move such an expensive and high quality service in the near future, we believe it should be closely linked to a hospital providing a full range of child health services.

We therefore recommend that:

1. The links between St George's Hospital and the Royal Marsden Hospital (Sutton) should be strengthened.

2. Child health services should be integrated within one clinical directorate.

In the longer term we recommend that paediatric oncology services should be transferred to either St George's Hospital or Guy's Hospital/St Thomas' Hospital, where they would link up with the paediatric oncology services transferred from St Bartholomew's Hospital. The aim would be to provide a single centre to serve the South East Thames and South West Thames regions.

St George's Hospital

Profile

St George's Hospital has a maternity unit, a neonatal intensive care unit and a paediatric intensive care unit. Its other services are paediatric neurology, paediatric immunology and infectious diseases, and it has interests in leukaemia, rheumatology and metabolic disease. Paediatric surgery has recently been transferred from Queen Mary's Hospital, Carshalton, which is scheduled for closure. Further detail is given in Appendix 2.

Commentary

St George's Hospital provides a full range of child health services at secondary level and a number of tertiary services. In our view it provides a sound base on which to build tertiary services. We recommend that:

1. The existing links between St George's Hospital and the Royal Marsden Hospital (Sutton) should be strengthened. Management arrangements should be integrated and child health services should be combined within one clinical directorate.

2. St George's Hospital should be considered as one of the sites for the transfer of paediatric oncology services from St Bartholomew's Hospital and, in the longer term, from the Royal Marsden Hospital (Sutton).

3. The St George's Trust and Wandsworth HA should satisfy themselves that the paediatric support for the care of children at Atkinson Morley is satisfactory.

6.6:   North West Sector

The district health authorities in this sector are the purchasing authorities for people living in the inner London boroughs of the City of Westminster, the Royal Borough of Kensington and Chelsea, and the London Borough of Hammersmith and Fulham. The total resident population of this sector is 723,000. It has a child population of 122,000 (16.9%).

The hospitals in this sector are:

- Charing Cross Hospital.
- Chelsea and Westminster Hospital.
- The Hammersmith Hospital.
- The Royal Brompton Hospital.
- St Mary's Hospital.

The Tomlinson report estimated the "exclusive population" of Charing Cross Hospital as 115,139 adults and children, and of St Mary's Hospital as 132,380 adults and children.

Note: The present number of providers of child health services in this sector, and the somewhat fragmented nature of the service they provide, suggests to us that a review should be undertaken by the principal purchasers in conjunction with the local providers to determine how the full range of child health services might best be delivered to the local populations. We believe the current pattern of service at this level may not meet the needs of the local populations and that services should be concentrated in fewer units which in turn should provide outreach services on a contractual basis.

In our opinion one outcome of such a review might be that St Mary's Hospital should assume responsibility for staffing the children's back-up ward for the accident and emergency department, or the servicing of outpatient and day care facilities, on the Hammersmith Hospital site.

Charing Cross Hospital

Commentary

The future of this hospital is in some doubt. Children's services were to be resited completely on closure of the A&E department. Whatever the outcome of consultation on the closure of the A&E department at Charing Cross the hospital does not meet our criteria as a centre for tertiary services. We do not recommend that any tertiary services for children are provided at the Charing Cross Hospital.

Chelsea and Westminster Hospital

Profile

The Chelsea and Westminster Hospital is a new hospital; it opened in 1993 on the site of the old St Stephen's Hospital. It has 45 children's beds, paediatric intensive care and neonatal intensive care, plus a full range of child health services, paediatric surgery, and with tertiary care in the fields of paediatric neurology and paediatric gastroenterology. All facilities meet the very latest standards for children's services. As this hospital is so new, there are likely to be changes in patient flow patterns that have yet to be established. Geographically, it is situated close to the Royal Brompton Hospital.

When we visited this hospital we were shown the ward to which the children's services would be transferred after the accident and emergency department at Charing Cross Hospital is closed. This proposal is the subject of consultation at present. Further detail is given in Appendix 2.

Commentary

Providing the management of the Chelsea and Westminster Hospital and the Royal Brompton Hospital are integrated and children's services are brought together under one clinical directorate, we recommend that the Royal Brompton Hospital should be considered as one of the options for the second cardiothoracic unit to serve the four Thames regions.

We consider the strength of this hospital to lie in its desire to provide high quality services to its local population. Since the Chelsea and Westminster Hospital has a bigger paediatric service than St Mary's Hospital, we recommend that this site should be developed as the centre for paediatric surgery for the North West Sector.

The Hammersmith Hospital

Profile

The Hammersmith Hospital has 20 children's beds, a maternity unit, a neonatal intensive care unit and an accident and emergency department. At tertiary level it provides a neuromuscular service, a haematology service (with facilities for bone marrow transplants), and a small paediatric medical and surgical service. It is planning to transfer the rheumatology service from Northwick Park Hospital, thereby extending the number of beds to 45. The neonatal paediatricians cover the Hammersmith Hospital and Queen Charlotte's Hospital and fetal medicine and obstetric medicine are strong. Further detail is given in Appendix 2.

Commentary

The Hammersmith Hospital does not provide a full range of child health services at secondary level and therefore does not meet our criteria for a tertiary centre. The services it does provide for the local population are limited.

The strength of this hospital lies in its academic and research work (and this is clearly its area of greatest interest judging from its "mission statement").

We did not feel that the tertiary services for children provided at the Hammersmith Hospital were complementary to each other. We therefore recommend that:

1. The neuromuscular service should be transferred to Great Ormond Street Hospital.

2.   Further consideration should be given to the most appropriate location for the transfer of the rheumatology service from Northwick Park Hospital. Once again, Great Ormond Street Hospital seems like the most appropriate location for this national service.

3.   Paediatric surgery in this sector should be provided at the Chelsea and Westminster Hospital.

4.   We recommend that the requirements for local children's services currently met by the Hammersmith Hospital might appropriately be provided on an out-reach basis from a hospital with a full range of child health services, such as St Mary's.

The Royal Brompton Hospital

Profile

The Royal Brompton Hospital is the second largest centre for cardiology and cardiothoracic work in south-east England. It serves an area of north west and south west London and takes patients from even further afield. It has extensive outreach clinics in a number of locations. The hospital provides a single specialty service (including academic and research work) in purpose-built accommodation of a high standard.

We heard from the hospital about its desire to develop links with the Chelsea and Westminster Hospital and St Mary's Hospital through its academic links with Imperial College. Further detail is given in Appendix 2.

Commentary

As a single-specialty hospital, the Royal Brompton Hospital does not provide a full range of child health services and therefore does not meet our criteria for a tertiary centre. However, due to its location, this problem can to an extent be overcome by integrating the management of the Chelsea and Westminster Hospital and the Royal Brompton Hospital and placing children's services at the two hospitals under the control of one clinical director. If this recommendation is implemented, the Royal Brompton Hospital should be considered as an option for the second paediatric cardiology and cardiothoracic centre in London, although the disadvantage of split site working would persist.

St Mary's Hospital

Profile

St Mary's Hospital has 22 general paediatric beds, 16 children's beds for infectious diseases including a small PICU, and 12 day care beds. It has a maternity unit and it provides a paediatric medical service and a paediatric surgical service. At tertiary level it provides infectious diseases, immunology and HIV services, and a paediatric neurology service. Further detail is given in Appendix 2.

Commentary

St Mary's provides a good children's service to the local population and, in addition, as a well developed infectious disease service. Its services are complementary to those at the Chelsea and Westminster although we believe that the latter should be the base for paediatric surgery in this sector.

The outpatient and daycare requirements for the local services at the Hammersmith could be provided from St Mary's.

Section 7: Strategic commissioning and the market

Contents of this section

7.1: OVERVIEW

Our model of care for tertiary services includes outreach clinics and shared management arrangements. It requires the tertiary centre to help in staff development at primary and secondary levels when necessary, and it requires hospitals to co-operate so that parents and children can retain their confidence in the ability of staff to provide the necessary care at every level.

For comparisons to be valid the clinical outcome of different hospitals must be compared on the basis of the results achieved against the population served, not on the basis of the results achieved in hospital.

For these reasons we believe tertiary services should have contractual arrangements with a defined catchment area — for example, the entire population covered by a district health authority. Reasons for referrals outside these contractual arrangements should be recorded or covered by a protocol. We did not find this to be the case at present.

We recognise that this model of care takes time to establish. <u>We therefore recommend</u> that contracts for children's tertiary services should be let for a period of more than one year.

Our recommendations ensure that purchasers have a choice of tertiary centre available for all but the most specific conditions with very low numbers of new cases per annum. They also mean that any hospital with a full range of child health services and an adult specialty at tertiary level will be able to come into the market with a children's specialty in that field if it can attract sufficient work. We are therefore satisfied that a proper balance has been struck between the need for competition and the delivery of an appropriate quality of service for children.

It is fundamental to our thinking that the principle of strategic commissioning outlined in the Audit Commission's report, **Children first**, will be followed. If the aim of delivering appropriate care in the right place at the right time is to be achieved, district health authorities which commission services from providers at secondary and tertiary levels will need to play an active role in co-ordinating services, or consider contracting out this role to one of their providers.

Our discussions with purchasers suggested that their priority would be to develop children's services at primary and secondary level. The development of specifications for each tertiary service might appropriately be handled on a consortium basis.

Our recommendations should result in the decentralisation on a shared care and outreach basis of all those elements of care which do not require the specialist investigation or treatment facilities of a tertiary centre; they will not result in a decentralisation of these facilities from inner London. (We concluded that to decentralise would actually reduce the competition and the choice available in the Thames regions.)

7.2: COSTS

In **Children first** the Audit Commission estimated that children account for about 10% of total expenditure on hospital and community health services. Although far fewer children come into contact with secondary and tertiary care than with primary care, the average costs of treating them is much greater.

We have had difficulty in identifying these costs. The financial returns did not provide information on the costs of tertiary services for children in the main specialities under review. We examined the possibility of using prices as an alternative but concluded that the variation from year to year and the variety of practices adopted made this a poor indicator and rendered such an approach invalid. Appendix 3 gives a summary of prices from ten providers.

Some examples of the different practices include:

- Different ways of treating costs for day cases, out-patients and overnight stays.

- Different descriptions of specialties.

- Different "currencies" (per day, per admission, per completed consultant episode).

- Lack of differentiation between prices for adults and prices for children.

We suggest that as a minimum costing standards as identified in EL(93)26 should be based on actual costs, costs should be established on a full cost basis, and that there should be no planned cross substitution between specialties, procedures or contracts.

In addition the guidance recommends that costs should be allocated directly to specialties where possible and specialties are defined on the same basis as in the Financial Return FR22 for the purposes of cost allocation and apportionment. Paediatrics are defined as a specialty in this return identifying actual activity and costs.

This approach should, if implemented by all providers start to ensure comparisons can be made between different providers and enable changes in expenditure on health services for children to be monitored.

7.3:   ACTIVITY

Our information on activity was obtained from a number of different sources:

- **From the North West Thames Management Information Unit** which analysed information on the five main specialty reviews for the first contracting year (1991-92) on behalf of the four Thames regions.

- **From hospitals providing tertiary services** who sent an "off-load" of their 1991/92 patient administration database to a central bureau for processing.

- **From provider units** who sent us their own information in their submissions to this review (unfortunately, the actual year covered in these submissions was variable).

- **From sources such as the British Paediatric Association** and **the Cancer Registration Centre.**

The information varied greatly in quality. Some of the identified shortcomings were:

- Some failure to code healthy babies. This was misleading and can lead to the exaggeration of the number of paediatric general medical episodes recorded.

- A failure to use specialty codes. This led to a failure to identify the workload of tertiary specialties.

- Variations on clinical practice. This led to quite different ratios between cases and episodes in different units.

In circumstances where there was an inexplicable difference between the various sources of information, we relied more on the data in the providers' own submissions.

7.4: MANPOWER

We have not attempted a detailed review of manpower. We have, however, set out in Table 8 at the end of this section, a comparison between the British Paediatric Association's recommendations on clinical manpower and our own assessment of the numbers of paediatric specialists in post (derived from the providers' own submissions).

Whilst concentrating on tertiary services will, in our view, improve the quality and standards of care for children, the scope for savings on medical staff seemed to us to be minimal or non-existent. This is partly due to the amount of clinical cover provided by academic staff: in one hospital, for example, none of the 7.5 full-time equivalent senior medical staff were employed by the hospital itself. Assuming standard conventions apply to the costing of contracts, this would mean that only the costs of their merit awards would be passed through into provider prices.

TABLE 8

CONSULTANT STAFFING NUMBERS

Specialty	BPA Recommended Consultant Staffing Level
Oncology	2 (Royal Marsden) 2 Barts 4 HSC
Nephrology	3 per Centre
Cardiology	No recommendation
Haematology	No recommendation
Complex Disability	2 per Region
Endocrinology	5 posts for London
Gastroenterology	2 per Region
Immunology	6 centres in UK each with 2
Infectious Diseases	2 per Region
Metabolic	2 per Region
Neurology	1 per 1m total population
Perinatal	Regional Centres 3
Respiratory	1.5-3 posts per Region
Rheumatology	1 per Region
Paediatric Surgery	No recommendation

Paediatric Units (Secondary Level) Based on birth rate	BPA Recommended Staffing Level
2000 or less	4 *
2000 - 3000	5 *
3000 - 4500 (without NIC)	6-7
3000 - 4500 (with NIC)	8
4500 - 6000	9-10

Numbers in post not assessed

Section 8: Summary of main conclusions and recommendations

Contents of this section

Section 8: **Summary of main conclusions and recommendations**

Main conclusions

Our analysis indicates that the child population of inner London is relatively deprived compared to children elsewhere in the four Thames regions. Evidence we have found from studies elsewhere indicate that at high levels of deprivation there may be difficulty in gaining access to healthcare. This issue needs to be addressed by inner London purchasers and providers (**section 2.2**).

It is our view that local service needs should not be given second place to the development of tertiary services. There are particular issues here for the north east sector (**section 6.3**).

There are currently eighteen hospital sites in inner London providing inpatient facilities for children at secondary care level. Given the high density population of an inner city, a hospital providing a full range of child health services might serve a local population of up to 300-500,000 with appropriately sited outpatient and daycare facilities off-site.

Even allowing for the relatively high use of hospital services by deprived populations, the requirements of inner London for high quality child health services at secondary care level could, in our view, be met by eight to ten inpatient hospitals each providing a full range of child health services (**section 2.3**).

We believe that there is an urgent need for purchasers in the Thames regions to decide how they are going to ensure a full range of child health services is available to their residents (**section 3**).

This issue is highly relevant to our recommendations for three reasons:

- Firstly, we conclude the tertiary services should only be based at hospitals that can provide a full range of child health services (**section 4.3**).

- Secondly, we are of the view that specialist children's services will not develop through an exclusive focus on each of the bodies major systems. Single specialty hospitals will therefore no longer be appropriate (**section 3.2**).

- Thirdly, we believe that a hospital providing a full range of child health services and hospitals providing tertiary services share a need for access to specific services such as paediatric intensive care and that larger paediatric intensive care units make better use of both specialist skills and are better able to absorb fluctuations in the workload (**section 5.6**).

Taking full account of all the advice received from reports, parents, professionals, consumer groups and voluntary agencies, we reached the following conclusions about the siting of tertiary services in London. These conclusions form the basis for our proposed changes to the pattern of service set out in section 6 of this report.

- A hospital that aims to provide tertiary services for children should first establish a full range of child health services for the local population.

- Tertiary services should not be moved to a hospital until that hospital is able to provide a full range of child health services for the local population.

- Tertiary services should be centred in a hospital, but should reach out to the whole population they serve.

- Access to tertiary services is a minor consideration when inpatient admission is required during the course of treatment. Most families are primarily concerned with the quality of the service and the outcome of the treatment.

- The mechanism for dealing with the dynamics of a tertiary service should be the contracting process between purchasers and providers at the primary/secondary and secondary/tertiary level interfaces.

- The outreach services provided by a tertiary centre should be based on a purchasing strategy that reflects the health needs of local children, rather than on history, tradition or personal contact. In this way tertiary centres will be able to support primary and secondary services in influencing the health of deprived populations in their vicinity.

- Tertiary centres should develop shared management arrangements to help with the "transfer of trust" from major centres to local services.

- Relocating services in London will require the highest level of skill. Parents fear that failure to manage change properly will result in a loss in the quality of care for their children.

In the light of our views on the location of tertiary services and access to them for the purposes of investigation and inpatient treatment we take the view that purchasers and providers should examine carefully how any inhibition that parents might have about travelling to a tertiary centre in inner London, due to the cost of such travel, should be overcome (**section 4.1**).

We recommend:

- that tertiary level inpatient services for children with cancer should be concentrated in two or three centres (section 5.1);

- that inpatient cardiology and cardiothoracic services at tertiary level in London should be concentrated in two or possibly three centres; (section 5.2)

- that tertiary paediatric neurology and neurosurgery services should be concentrated in two or possibly three tertiary centres; (section 5.3)

- that paediatric nephrology be provided in two centres; (section 5.4)

- that specialist plastic surgery be concentrated on two or three centres; (section 5.5)

- that there should be five paediatric surgical centres in London providing a specialist paediatric surgery and neonatal surgery. (section 5.6)

We have concluded that:

- the Hospital for Sick Children, Great Ormond Street does not, in its current configuration, meet our criteria for a tertiary centre in that it does not provide a full range of child health services for a local population.

We recommend that:

- these deficiencies be overcome by building on the Government's initiative announced in '**Making London better**' through integration with the University College/Middlesex and Great Ormond Street.

- this process is further developed through links between Great Ormond Street and the Royal Free Hospital and/or the Whittington Hospital.

- subject to the above, Great Ormond Street should continue to build on its role as a major tertiary centre providing the full range of tertiary services including cancer, cardiology and cardiothoracic services, neurology and neurosurgical services, nephrology services, plastic surgery, specialist paediatric surgery, and other specialty services.

- the neuromuscular service currently at the Hammersmith Hospital, the rheumatology service currently at Northwick Park and the retinoblastoma service currently at St Bartholomew's should, subject to proper facilities being made available for them, be considered for transfer to Great Ormond Street.

- the Guy's or St Thomas' site should be a second major centre including the provision of paediatric nephrology and paediatric neuroscience services.

- contracts for children's tertiary services should be let for a period of more than one year. (**section 4**)

We suggest that:

- the advice given in recent official guidance on costing standards should be met as quickly as possible. (**section 7**)

During our Review we have had the benefit of the views, advice and information from a wide range of individuals and organisations. This information, not all of which can be incorporated into the report, could be of considerable use to those who have to assess and implement our advice. We shall be pleased to make it available.

We believe that our advice will produce a sound basis for education and research as well as health services for the future. Although we have concentrated on the location of tertiary services in inner London the implementation of our recommendations would build close contractual links between the hospitals providing the base for tertiary services and the populations that they serve in the Thames regions.

Section 9: Executive Summary

Contents of this section

Section 9: Executive summary

9.1 Introduction

Purpose of the Review

The purpose of the speciality reviews was set out in Making London Better.

> **For each speciality, the review groups will assess current and projected needs, define appropriate models of care and criteria for tertiary centres and develop a service specification. They will advise on an appropriate pattern of service the speciality and on where departments should be located cost-effectively to achieve the best clinical outcome. The work will be co-ordinated and supported by LIG and options developed for Ministers' decisions by the end of May. These reports may, in some cases, lead to the modification of the general proposals for change to acute services set out later in this document.**

Coverage and strategic commissioning

We believe tertiary services should have contractual links to cover a defined catchment area. Our recommendations ensure that there will be a choice of tertiary centres available for all but the most specific conditions with very low numbers of new cases per annum.

It is fundamental to our thinking that the principle of strategic commissioning outlined in the Audit Commission's Report Children First will be followed. If the aim of delivering the appropriate care in the right place at the right time is to be followed, District Health Authorities commissioning care from more than one provider will need to play an active role in co-ordinating services unless they contract this role to one of their providers.

We therefore make no distinction between Inner and Outer London or the rest of the Thames Regions when referring to the need for outreach clinics, shared care arrangements or contractual relationships between tertiary and secondary care.

Our recommendations should result in decentralisation on a shared care and outreach basis of all those elements of care which do not require the specialist investigation or treatment facilities of the tertiary centre. They will not result in the decentralisation of these facilities from Inner London, since we have concluded that to decentralise would actually reduce the competition and choice available within the Thames Regions.

Map of hospitals

The location hospitals to which we refer are shown on the map at Appendix 1.

9.2   The model of care

Principles

We were advised by many, and it is government policy, that children in hospital must be cared for in an environment sensitive to their needs and by people trained in their care. We have taken the view that all speciality services must be based on hospitals with a full range of children's health services. We agree that many who argued that children's services should not be part of a 'single organ' speciality hospital.

We believe that in the context of London, a full range of children's health services should at secondary level consist of:

- An A&E service with a separate admission space for children.

- A paediatric medical service.

- A paediatric surgical service.

- Maternity services with neonatal intensive care.

- A children's intensive care service [paediatric intensive care].

- Children's support services, therapists, teachers, etc.

- A home nursing service, and a parent care approach.

We accept that these standards may not be appropriate universally, but believe they can and should be obtained in London due to the high density of the population.

Population size: secondary and tertiary services

Secondary Care Services

In the language of the moment it should be a child and family focused services. Any hospital serving a population in London of 500,000, with a birth rate of approximately 6000, should have a full range of these services. In areas of deprivation a population of 300,000 with birthrates over 3,500 would justify a similar range of services. Hospitals serving smaller populations may elect to send infants needing neonatal intensive care, children requiring intensive care and paediatric surgery to an adjacent hospital.

Tertiary Specialist Services

Whatever the population served, tertiary services should be based on a hospital with a full range of child health services.

Outreach

The service should be closely linked with the population it serves. The aim has always been that a child should be admitted to hospital only when there is no other alternative. We expect each speciality service to serve a specific catchment population and to have outreach clinics and outreach services, as appropriate to the speciality.

As the full range of children's health services is developed throughout the Thames Regions and as shortages of consultant paediatric staffing are overcome, we would expect shared care to develop and the tertiary centres to transfer back to the secondary care centre.

In other words, a service should be delivered to the child and not the child to the service.

Becoming adult

Each service should have clearly described routes by which a child with a disease or disorder that persists into adolescence and young adulthood will be provided with care appropriate to their changing circumstances.

Access

We discussed the issue of access at length, and raised it as a question with the provider units, with purchasers and with voluntary organisations.

On the basis of the model of care which we are advocating and the small numbers of children suffering from each condition per 100,00 children in the population, we have concluded that access/travelling time to the tertiary centre is not a critical factor, providing proper outreach and shared care arrangements are in place and children are not brought to the tertiary centre for purposes other than clinical care.

We did take the view that it was essential to have two or more tertiary centres in order to give purchasers acting in conjunction with other groups within their local population, a choice of centre.

We are however, aware that some parents may be unable to afford the costs of travel to a tertiary centre and believe this issue should be addressed to ensure that no children are disadvantaged by virtue of the cost of travel to their family.

Conclusion

The position we have therefore taken is:-

    a. Hospitals which aim to provide tertiary services should first aim to provide a full range of child health services for their local population.

    b. Tertiary services should not be moved to hospitals until they are able to provide a full range of services to the local population.

    c. Tertiary services have a centre in a hospital but reach out to the whole population they serve.

9.3 Summary of the main recommendations and options

From analyses and from the advice we received from specialists, we formed the view that the child population of South East England would be best served by the following number of speciality units:

Speciality	Recommended Number of Sites
Cardiac Services	2/3
Neurosciences	2/3
Nephrology	2
Oncology	2
Plastics	2

The Hospitals for Sick Children will be one of the centres for each speciality. **Guy's or St Thomas'**, depending on the site chosen, could become the second major centre with a wide range of tertiary services.

Cardiac services for children

We recommend that:

a. In-patient cardiothoracic centres be concentrated on two sites.

b. One of these centres should be the **Hospital for Sick Children/Great Ormond Street.**

c. The other centre be either **Guy's/St Thomas'** or **The Royal Brompton** with **The Chelsea & Westminster.**

d. A precondition of the **Royal Brompton/Chelsea and Westminster** option would be the integration of the management of these two units with children's services becoming the responsibility of one clinical director across the combined unit.

e.   Subject to the above precondition being acted upon, an acceptable alternative would be the use of three units, **Hospital for Sick Children/Great Ormond Street, Royal Brompton/Chelsea and Westminster** and **Guy's/St Thomas'**.

f.   In our view, children should no longer be admitted to **Harefield Hospital**.

Neurology and neurosurgery

We recommend that:-

a.   There should be two or three in-patient centres at tertiary level for neurology and neurosurgery.

b.   These centres should also be secondary level centres for neurological services for children and head injury services.

c.   **Hospital for Sick Children** should be one of the centres.

d.   **Guy's/St Thomas'** should be the second centre.

e.   **Atkinson Morley's Hospital** should cease to admit children once the second neurosciences centre is established on the **Guy's/St Thomas'** site.

We further advise:-

f.   That until the **Guy's/St Thomas'** centre is established, **St. George's Healthcare NHS Trust** should ensure that there is a satisfactory paediatric input into the care of children treated at **Atkinson Morley.**

g.   We would keep open the option for the establishment of a third neurosciences in-patient centre for children until we know the outcome of the adult neurosciences review.

h.   Other centres, such as **The Royal London** or the centre to which **Atkinson Morley** is finally located could also open up an in-patient neurosciences services at tertiary level providing they have comprehensive child health services on site and an adult service in the speciality.

Nephrology

We recommend that:-

a.   There should be two centres for paediatric nephology, one should be at the **Hospital for Sick Children** linked with the **Royal Free or University College/Middlesex** dependent on the establishment of adult services, and the other at **Guy's/St Thomas'**.

Cancer services

We recommend that:-

a.   Two large paediatric oncology units be formed in the long term.

b.   One of these units should be based on a joint unit between **University College Hospital/Middlesex** and **The Hospitals For Sick Children**. The location of the second unit will depend on the outcome of the adult review but may be either at **Guy's/St Thomas'** or **St George's**.

We recommend that in the interim:-

c.   One clinical directorate should be responsible for the management of all the children's services within the **St Bartholomew's/Royal London**.

d.   Management responsibility for **The Royal Marsden Hospital (Sutton)** should be merged with **St George's Healthcare Trust** and that one clinical directorate should be responsible for children's services within **St George's** and **Royal Marsden (Sutton)**.

General recommendations

We recommend:

- All children's specialist services should develop a model of care based on close and appropriate links between the tertiary centre and the population served. Only those procedures which must be undertaken at the tertiary centre should be centralised. There should be a contractual relationship between the tertiary centre and the secondary care centres which it services.

Plastic surgery and burns

We are advised that plastic surgery is seen as a secondary care service.

We recommend:-

a. That for that element of plastic surgery which works in conjunction with specialists at tertiary level (e.g. cranio-facial surgery) there should be two centres, one based on the **Hosital for Sick Children/University College** complex and one elsewhere.

We are unable to advise:-

b. On the location of the second centre or on burns units until we have seen a summary of the adult review.

Paediatric surgery

We recommend:-

a. Paediatric surgery be developed in five teams, with each team having responsibility for paediatric surgery in a particular area of London.

We recommend that the basis for the five teams should be:-

b.   **The Royal London** to which the paediatric surgical service from **Queen Elizabeth Hospital** should be transferred.

c.   **St. George's Hospital NHS Trust.**

d.   **The Chelsea & Westminster Hospital.**

e.   **The Hospitals for Sick Children.**

f.   The service in the South East sector is currently based at **Lewisham Hospital.** The centre of activity may shift depending on the siting of tertiary services. No conclusion yet reached.

9.4   Sector and unit analysis

In this section we review the services currently available and identify actions required to create the full range of child health services upon which tertiary services should be based.

It seemed to us that the medical schools and special health authorities fall into five territories, and that these are linked with district general hospitals which service local or adjacent populations. These five sectors are:

The North Central Sector
The North East Sector
The South East Sector
The South West Sector
The North West Sector

The north central sector

The health authority in this sector of Inner London is responsible for the populations of Bloomsbury, Islington and Hampstead. The total resident population of this area is 348,000 with a child population of 69,000 (19.9%). Sited within that area is the **UCH/Middlesex; the Royal Free; the Whittington; the**

Whittington; The Hospitals for Sick Children (GOS) and the **Hospital for Nervous Diseases.**

The number of births at the **UCH/Middlesex** and **The Royal Free,** and the number of general paediatric medical admissions at these units, does not suggest that they are individually serving a population of the size we would expect in an Inner City area, nor sufficient to justify a full range of services for children.

The Hospitals for Sick Children

The **HSC** provides a very extensive range of tertiary services for children in the Thames Regions; undertakes a significant amount of work for other regions; is a national centre with a number of supra-regional services; undertakes international work by providing tertiary services for countries not large enough to establish them for themselves, and undertakes research and development work on its own account and in conjunction with the **Institute of Child Health.**

The services provided by **The Hospitals for Sick Children** is deficient in a number of important areas. It lacks an A&E Department; it does not have a maternity or neonatal medical service, and it has limited services for adolescents and arbitrary associations with speciality services for adults.

To meet our criteria for a tertiary centre **Hospital for Sick Children** must overcome these deficiencies and we have looked at ways this can be accomplished.

It is therefore essential to any plan for tertiary services in London that **Hospital for Sick Children** makes a smooth transition into the market environment and finds ways of overcoming its current deficiencies.

We recommend that:

      a.   the Hospital for Sick Children should provide secondary level service to its local population in conjunction with other local units.

             There are a number of ways in which integration into a local population can be achieved and these options will be set out in the full report.

We advise:-

b.   That both the **University College/Middlesex** and **The Royal Free Hospital** are too small to support a secondary service. In our view neither should continue to have in-patient services for children.

We recommend:

c.   That **University College/Middlesex** and **Royal Free** concentrate on the provision of services for adolescents and adults with **Hospital for Sick Children** admitting all children below a certain age requiring secondary care services.

We advise:

d.   That this arrangement is particularly attractive with respect to oncology services, since it would involve bringing together two of the London UKCCSG centres for cancer to provide a comprehensive service for children with cancer from infancy to young adulthood.

The University College and Middlesex Hospitals

University College has excellent maternity, fetal and neonatal services and a strong science base. It provides a relatively small service in terms of general paediatric admissions.

We recommend:

That it should link its paediatric services with **Hospital for Sick Children** and concentrate on providing a quality out-patient and daycase centre either without in-patient responsibilities or with the level required to support only the A&E.

The Royal Free Hospital

This hospital has developed a community oriented child health service but provides a relatively small service in terms of general paediatric admissions.

We recommend:

    a.   That it should link its paediatric services with HSC and concentrate on providing a quality out-patient centre and community services, either without in-patient responsibilities or with the level required to support only A&E.

We suggest:

    b.   It should provide tertiary adolescent facilities depending on which tertiary services are placed there.

We further suggest:

    c.   From the perspective of children's services, that consideration might be given to the appropriate management arrangements between **University College/Middlesex** the **Royal Free** and **Hospital for Sick Children**.

The north east sector

The health authority in this sector of Inner London is responsible for the population of the City & Hackney, Newham and Tower Hamlets. The residents population of this area is 569,400 with a child population of 135,650 (23.85). The proportion of the children in the population is the highest in Inner London, and the level of deprivation is also high.

The first priority is to provide a full range of services for children to the local population.

Sited within that area are **The Homerton Hospital, Newham Hospital, Queen Elizabeth Hospital, The Royal London Hospital** and **St Bartholomew's Hospital**.

Neither **The Homerton, The Royal London** nor **St Bartholomew's Hospital** provide a full range of services for children at present. **St Bartholomew's Hospital** does not itself have a sufficient local population to support one. Nor, given the configuration of hospitals around it , can this be achieved.

The Queen Elizabeth Hospital provides a valued service to the local population but cannot remain indefinitely on its present site.

We recommend that:

a. No tertiary services are placed on any site in this sector until a full range of services for children is established to meet the high level of need in the local population.

b. **Queen Elizabeth Hospital** is moved to the **Royal London Hospital** site to create a unit with a full range of child health services at secondary care level.

c. The tertiary services at **Barts NHS Trust** are transferred elsewhere in due course, the preferred options being - retinoblastoma to **Hospital for Sick Children** as it is a national service paediatric oncology either to **Guy's/St Thomas'** or to **St George's** to link up with the **Royal Marsden** services (these options are dependent of the outcome of the adult reviews).

d. Requirements of the local population in relation to outreach out-patient and daycare services at both secondary and tertiary level be reviewed to determine requirements for services at **The Homerton** the current **Queen Elizabeth** site and the **St Bartholomew's** site.

e. The **Queen Elizabeth (Hackney)/Royal London** should establish an ambulatory paediatric service and cover arrangements for the maternity and neonatal services at **the Homerton Hospital**.

South east sector

The health authority in this sector of inner London is responsible for the population of West Lambeth, Camberwell, Lewisham and North Southwark. The total resident population is 707,000 with a child population of 139,000 (19.6%). There are five provider units at present, **Guys Hospital, Kings Hospital, Lewisham Hospital, Maudsley Hospital and St Thomas' Hospital.**

Service provision for the local population does not appear to be co-ordinated or complementary. We prefer **King's College Hospital** as a potential site for tertiary services, since it has a sensitive approach to the care of the child within a full range of child health services. However, it was not favoured by the adult reviews.

We recommend:

a. Paediatric neurosciences be established on the **Guy's/St Thomas'** site.

b.   The **Guy's/St Thomas'** site be considered as one of the options for the relocation of the paediatric oncology service currently provided at **St Bartholomew's Hospital.**

c.   Paediatric nephrology services remain on the **Guy's/St Thomas'** site.

d.   Providing the conditions of our option for cardiothoracic services are met, one option is the transfer of cardiac services to **The Royal Brompton Hospital.**

Our recommendations for the transfer of oncology services and neuroscience services to the **Guy's/St Thomas'** site will put pressure on whichever is chosen, and the recommendations of the adult service reviews may add to this pressure. We believe careful assessment of the overall site plan and costs are required before final decisions are made.

We further suggest:

e.   A local review of child health service be undertaken.

South west sector

The Health Authority in this sector of inner London is responsible for the population of part of Wandsworth. The total resident population is 191,200 with a child population of 34,000 (17.8%). **St. George's Hospital** is the only unit physically located within that population, and it is sited at the southern boundary.

We recommend:

a.   The links between **St George's** and the **Royal Marsden (Sutton)** should be strengthened, with **St George's** taking management responsibility for **The Royal Marsden (Sutton).** Child health services should be within one clinical directorate.

b.   As soon as a neurosciences centre for children is established at **Guy's/St Thomas'** children should cease to be admitted to **Atkinson Morley.** In the meantime the paediatric input to the service for children at **Atkinson Morley** should be strengthened.

We further recommend that:

    c.   The review of acute services set up as a result of **Making London Better** should consider whether the local population is best served by so many separate paediatric in-patient centres.

The north west sector

The health authority in this sector of Inner London were Riverside and Parkside. Together they had a total resident population of 723,000 with a child population of 122,000 (16.9%). Sited within this area are **The Charing Cross Hospital, The Chelsea & Westminster Hospital, The Hammersmith & Queen Charlotte's Hospitals,** and **St. Mary's Hospital.**

Children's services at the **Charing Cross Hospital** are due to transfer to **The Chelsea & Westminster Hospitals** on the closure of the A&E Department at **Charing Cross.** However, this proposal is currently subject to consultation.

We recommend that:-

    a.   The Hammersmith Hospital should not continue to provide general in-patient services for children as the volume is too small to support a full range of child health services. There is the possibility of servicing their in-patient requirement with an outreach service from **St. Mary's Hospital.**

    b.   The service for children with muscular disorders be transferred from **The Hammersmith to Hospital for Sick Children.**

    c.   The rheumatology service which is due to be transferred from **Northwick Park Hospital** be transferred to Hospital for Sick Children or another unit where the full range of child health services is present (e.g. Chelsea & Westminster or St Mary's).

    d.   We recognise the benefit that children can derive from the considerable scientific expertise and research investment at **The Hammersmith Hospital** and suggest that the Research Departments at **The Hammersmith Hospital** approach **The Institute of Child Health** or other appropriate bodies to facilitate their access to sick children for research purposes.

e. **Chelsea & Westminster Hospital** and **St Mary's Hospital** have a wide range of services and the opportunity to develop tertiary services and shared care arrangements.

9.5 General recommendations

Finally, we make a general recommendation that purchasers review with their local primary and secondary care providers the current provision for children's services in their districts and determine how a full range of child health services might most effectively be developed to meet local requirements.

9.6 Education and research

The five sectors on which we have based our recommendations are consistent with the location of the five Medical School groupings being developed in London.

Our proposals should result in the establishment of a full range of child health services at secondary level in the area of each medical school grouping and concentrate tertiary services.

We believe these proposals will support not only undergraduate and postgraduate medical education and research, but also the education of the nurses and professional staff without whom the service will not reach the appropriate standards.

Child population in the four Thames Regions

Each Region plus DHAs, purchasing authorities, inner & outer London & the rest of Thames

North West Thames

DHAs		Total District Population	Births	Age Group (yrs.)				Population Projections 0 - 14 yrs	
				<1	1 - 4	5 - 14	Total 0 - 14	1989 based projection for 1993	percentage change in 2010 compared with 1993 data
Riverside	)Inner	290,507	3,879	3,829	12,206	23,120	39,155	45,255	3.65
Parkside	)London	432,571	6,667	6,729	21,471	48,077	76,277	76,724	3.21
Total		723,078	10,546	10,558	33,677	71,197	115,432		
Barnet	)	298,145	4,192	4,157	16,005	35,511	55,673	60,537	6.75
Harrow	)	202,924	2,779	2,815	10,726	25,231	38,772	39,644	10.89
Hillingdon	)Outer	235,231	3,602	3,515	13,080	27,683	44,278	47,732	6.77
Hounslow & Spelthorne	)London	299,086	4,349	4,422	16,127	34,767	55,316	57,517	7.50
Ealing	)	280,031	4,442	4,381	15,284	34,002	53,667	57,883	-3.01
Total		1,315,417	19,366	19,290	71,222	157,194	247,706		
N Bedfordshire	)	249,738	3,346	3,331	13,641	32,514	49,486	53,614	9.92
S Bedfordshire	)	248,806	4,783	4,892	18,228	39,636	62,756	64,853	3.10
E&N Hertfordshire	)rest of	483,659	6,674	6,665	26,267	59,717	92,649	E56,544 N38,031	-0.34 -0.51
NW Hertfordshire	)Thames	260,788	3,428	3,505	13,614	32,936	50,055	51,468	1.50
SW Hertfordshire	)	242,941	3,316	3,430	13,105	29,149	45,684	47,847	6.99
Total		1,521,932	21,547	21,823	84,855	193,952	300,630		
TOTAL				51,671	189,754	422,343	663,768		

North East Thames

DHAs	Total District Population	Births	Age Group (yrs.)				Population Projections 0 - 14	
			<1	1 - 4	5 - 14	Total	1989 based population projection for 1993	percentage change in 2010 compared with 1993 data
Hampstead)	105,000	1,294	1,300	4,500	10,000	15,800	17,194	-2.17
City & Hackney) Inner	187,400	3,829	3,800	12,400	25,100	41,300	44,292	-3.99
Newham) London	217,100	4,558	4,500	15,400	31,200	51,100	51,866	15.00
Tower Hamlets)	164,900	3,228	3,100	12,100	25,000	40,200	39,487	15.99
Bloomsbury & Islington)	242,500	3,752	3,800	13,100	25,600	42,500	Bl. 18,769 / Isl. 33,351	4.19 / -0.73
Total	916,900	16,661	16,500	57,500	116,900	190,900		
Enfield)	261,600	3,692	3,900	14,500	31,300	49,700	53,033	13.00
Haringey)	207,000	3,489	3,500	11,900	23,600	39,000	38,713	4.49
Redbridge) OL	230,000	3,335	3,400	12,100	27,900	43,400	43,322	13.18
Waltham Forrest) PA	215,800	3,856	3,800	12,700	25,600	42,100	44,921	0.05
Total	914,400	14,642	14,600	51,200	108,400	174,200		
Basildon & Thurrock)	291,900	4,399	4,400	17,300	38,300	60,000	58,124	-9.53
Mid Essex)	294,600	4,083	4,000	16,200	38,000	58,200	58,094	5.48
NE Essex) rest	306,800	3,748	3,800	15,200	35,300	54,300	59,969	26.06
West Essex)	259,000	3,348	3,300	13,400	31,300	48,000	48,913	-2.32
Southend)	326,300	4,184	4,200	16,300	39,200	59,700	60,629	-3.86
Barking, Havering & Brentwood)	447,400	5,994	6,000	23,800	54,300	84,100	84,021	-2.19
Total	1,926,000	25,756	25,700	102,200	236,400	364,300		
TOTAL			56,800	210,900	461,700	729,400		

South West Thames			Age Group (yrs.)					Population Projections 0 - 14	
DHAs		Total District Population	Births	<1	1 - 4	5 - 14	Total 0 - 14	1989 based projection for 1993	percentage change in 2010 compared with 1993 data
Wandsworth	Inner London	191,200	3,209	3,000	9,500	17,200	29,700	34,008	2.58
Merton & Sutton)		340,800	5,012	4,900	18,500	38,100	61,500	65,234	7.56
Croydon)		317,400	4,934	5,000	17,900	38,000	60,900	64,385	5.04
Kingston & Esher) OL		183,400	2,428	2,400	9,200	20,300	31,900	32,698	12.43
Richmond,)		230,900	2,978	3,000	1,100	23,100	27,200	42,751	20.36
Twickenham &)									
Roehampton)									
Total		1,072,500	15,352	15,300	46,700	119,500	181,500		
NW Surrey)		214,800	2,846	2,800	11,100	24,500	38,400	38,194	6.81
W Surrey &)		283,000	3,806	3,900	15,500	35,500	54,900	54,545	10.11
NE Hants)									
SW Surrey)		188,500	2,228	2,300	8,700	22,200	33,200	34,030	-4.72
Mid Surrey) rest		169,300	1,842	1,900	7,900	19,700	29,500	30,786	19.11
E Surrey)		190,400	2,353	2,300	5,400	22,300	30,000	34,197	19.11
Chichester)		179,700	1,866	2,000	7,700	19,100	28,800	30,043	6.72
Mid Downs)		285,700	3,746	3,800	15,000	36,800	55,600	55,512	19.73
Worthing)		248,300	2,727	2,800	11,300	26,300	40,400	40,953	8.37
									22.49
Total		1,759,700	21,414	21,800	82,600	206,400	310,800		
TOTAL				40,100	138,800	343,100	522,000		

South East Thames

DHAs		Total District Population	Births	Age Group (yrs.)				Population Projections 0 - 14 yrs	
				<1	1 -4	5 - 14	Total 0 - 14	1989 based population projection for 1993	percentage change in 2010 compared with 1993 data
W Lambeth	)PA	161,400	2,803	2,700	9,200	17,000	28,900	27,469	-0.84
Camberwell	)&	218,000	3,932	3,900	13,800	26,200	43,900	46,766	-6.24
Lewisham &	)IL	327,700	5,607	5,600	19,800	37,700	63,100	64,724	9.26
N Southwark	)								
Total		707,100	12,342	12,200	42,800	80,900	135,900		
Bexley	)PA	218,000	3,103	3,200	12,100	26,300	41,600	42,310	-3.52
Greenwich	)OL	211,900	3,552	3,500	13,200	27,700	44,400	47,150	18.77
Bromley	)	292,800	3,604	3,600	14,400	32,700	50,700	54,710	15.70
Total		722,700	10,259	10,300	39,700	86,700	136,700		
Brighton	)	310,900	3,698	3,700	14,900	31,200	48,900	51,200	10.40
Eastbourne	)	237,000	2,513	2,600	10,700	26,700	40,000	42,469	33.39
Hastings	)	168,600	2,020	2,000	8,100	19,000	29,100	30,466	16.81
SE Kent	)	273,600	3,559	3,600	14,200	32,800	50,600	54,134	15.27
Canterbury & Thanet	) rest of	303,400	3,645	3,700	14,700	35,600	54,000	58,012	10.33
Dartford & Gravesham	) Thames	223,000	3,085	3,100	12,400	27,700	43,200	40,971	-21.39
Maidstone	)	201,100	2,509	2,700	10,800	25,300	38,800	40,528	9.18
Medway	)	334,900	5,127	5,100	20,100	45,100	70,300	69,913	0.87
Tunbridge Wells	)	202,600	2,655	2,400	9,700	24,400	36,500	34,271	-14.10
Total		2,255,100	28,811	28,900	115,600	250,700	412,300		
TOTAL				51,400	198,100	418,300	667,800		

North West Thames DHAs	Percent heads of household from New Commonwealth and Pakistan	Population density/hectare
Riverside	8.7	90.1
Parkside	-	70.3
Barnet	9.2	33.3
Harrow	10.8	36.6
Hillingdon	4.8	21.3
Hounslow & Spelthorne	8	50.5
Ealing	17.0	
N Bedfordshire	3.7	
S Bedfordshire	6.2	
E&N Hertfordshire	3.2 & 1.5	
NW Hertfordshire	2.3	
SW Hertfordshire	2.9	

* England 0

● Relates to total population: 0-14 age group available

Source: Public Health Common Data set 1992

percent ethnic population from the 1991 census:-

Brent	44.8
City of Westminster	21.4
Harrow	26.2
Hounslow	24.4
Ealing	32.3

North East Thames DHAs	Percent heads of household from New Commonwealth and Pakistan	Population density/hectare
Hampstead	8.1	77.1
City & Hackney	20.6	84.3
Newham	17.5	59.7
Tower Hamlets	13.2	83.5
Bloomsbury & Islington	-	105.5
Enfield	10.2	32.2
Haringey	22.0	
Redbridge	7.5	40.7
Waltham Forest	11.4	54.4
Basildon & Thurrock	1.6	
Mid Essex	1.4	
NE Essex	1.3	
West Essex	1.6	
Southend	1.3	
Barking, Havering & Brentwood	2.0	14.9

percent ethnic population from the 1991 census:

Hackney	33.6
Newham	42.3
Tower Hamlets	35.6
Islington	18.9
Redbridge	21.4
Waltham Forest	25.6

South West Thames DHAs	Percent heads of household from New Commonwealth and Pakistan	Population density/hectare
Wandsworth	16.2	84.7
Merton & Sutton	5.5	41.9
Croydon	9.0	36.6
Kingston & Esher	3.9	27.5
Richmond, Twickenham & Roehampton	4.3	34.2
NW Surrey	2.4	
W Surrey & NE Hants	2.6	
SW Surrey	1.9	
Mid Surrey	2.1	
E Surrey	1.9	
Chichester	1.3	
Mid Downs	2.3	
Worthing	1.4	

percent ethnic population from the 1991 census:-

Wandsworth   20.0

South East Thames DHAs	Percent heads of household from New Commonwealth and Pakistan	Population density/hectare
W Lambeth	17.0	103.2
Camberwell	16.6	73.6
Lewisham & N Southwark	10.2	72.0
Bexley	3.1	36.0
Greenwich	5.7	44.4
Bromley	2.9	19.3
Brighton	2.0	
Eastbourne	1.5	
Hastings	1.4	
SE Kent	1.3	
Canterbury & Thanet	1.1	
Dartford & Gravesham	3.1	
Maidstone	1.4	
Medway	2.6	
Tunbridge Wells	1.6	

percent ethnic population from the 1991 census:-

Southwark   24.4

Lewisham   22.0

PROVIDER PROFILES AND ACTIVITY ANALYSIS

We do not guarantee the accuracy of the information contained in these profiles. However, they give a 'feel' for the size and range of services provided for children by the hospital.

The sources from which the data was extracted were:

Births	Latest data supplied to the BPA by RHAs in 1992
Paediatric General Medical FCE)	From providers PAS offload tapes.
)	
Tertiary specialty FCE)	Where no tape submitted Regional data has been
)	
Total FCEs 1991/92)	used instead. Information
)	processed by Price
)	Waterhouse NMR Bureau.
)	
Number of consultants/professors named	Extracted from provider submissions requires validation (see note in Section 7 re manpower)

NORTH EAST SECTOR

Hospital	Number of Births 1991	Number of Paediatric Medical FCE's (1) 1991/92 Code 420	Number of Tertiary Specialty FCE's (2) 1991/92	Total FCE's Children 1991/2 All Codes	Number of Consultants/ Professors Named	Average Length of Stay Comparison (3)
Newham	4072	2282				
St. Bartholomew's		1077	859	3547	6	4.10/2.91
Homerton	4014	149		461	2	6.74/3.33
Royal London	3357	1910	359	5358 (A)	4	4.00/2.89
Q E H		1860	2013	4799		

(1)   This information may include well babies

(2)   Tertiary Specialty FCE's Specialty Codes: 150, 110, 170, 171, 301, 302, 303, 320, 340, 350, 361, 370, 400, 421, 800, 823, 830

(3)   The first figures gives the average length of stay in the hospital in days for all paediatric FCE's. The second gives the comparison against all DRG codes taken into account on the database.

(A)   Includes 854 FCE's Code 501. (Obstetrics for patients using a bed)

NORTH CENTRAL SECTOR

Hospital	Number of Births 1991	Number of Paediatric Medical FCE's (1) 1991/92 Code 420	Number of Tertiary Specialty FCE's (2) 1991/92	Total FCE's Children 1991/2 All Codes	Number of Consultants/ Professors Named	Average Length of Stay Comparison (3)
Whittington	3055	3167		4585	3	3.41/2.89
Royal Free	2380	1701	1265	3778	7	3.82/2.93
UCH/Middlesex	3050	2230	465	3684	10	Note (A)
H S C		644	9566	14087	72	5.01/3.94

(1) This information may include well babies

(2) Tertiary Specialty FCE's Specialty Codes: 150, 110, 170, 171, 301, 302, 303, 320, 340, 350, 361, 370, 400, 421, 800, 823, 830

(3) The first figures gives the average length of stay in the hospital in days for all paediatric FCE's. The second gives the comparison against all DRG codes taken into account on the database.

(A) Average length of stay for 949 general paediatrics. FCE's 9.42 days compared to 3.55. Suggests error in figures or specialised workload.

NORTH WEST SECTOR

Hospital	Number of Births 1991	Number of Paediatric Medical FCE's (1) 1991/92 Code 420	Number of Tertiary Specialty FCE's (2) 1991/92	Total FCE's Children 1991/2 All Codes	Number of Consultants/ Professors Named	Average Length of Stay Comparison (3)
St Mary's	2600	2297	218	4126	8	3.97/2.85
Royal Brompton			1553	1553	4	4.58/5.61
Hammersmith	1200	2729	393	3321		6.10/3.15
Queen Charlotte's	4200				7.5	
Riverside Acute and Community Unit	2240	2661	1287	5823	8	3.65/2.86

(1)   This information may include well babies

(2)   Tertiary Specialty FCE's Specialty Codes: 150, 110, 170, 171, 301, 302, 303, 320, 340, 350, 361, 370, 400, 421, 800, 823, 830

(3)   The first figures gives the average length of stay in the hospital in days for all paediatric FCE's. The second gives the comparison against all DRG codes taken into account on the database.

SOUTH EAST SECTOR

Hospital	Number of Births 1991	Number of Paediatric Medical FCE's (1) 1991/92 Code 420	Number of Tertiary Specialty FCE's (2) 1991/92	Total FCE's Children 1991/2 All Codes	Number of Consultants/ Professors Named	Average Length of Stay Comparison (3)
King's	3775	2643	443	6384 (A)	9	2.72/2.84
St.Thomas / Guy's	6395	2250	3603	8769 (C)	20	St.T 3.32/2.88 Guy's 2.10/2.92
Lewisham (B) / Maudsley	2702	1953	1164	5049		1.71/2.88

(1) This information may include well babies

(2) Tertiary Specialty FCE's Specialty Codes: 150, 110, 170, 171, 301, 302, 303, 320, 340, 350, 361, 370, 400, 421, 800, 823, 830

(3) The first figures gives the average length of stay in the hospital in days for all paediatric FCE's. The second gives the comparison against all DRG codes taken into account on the database.

(A) Includes 2039 FCE's in oral surgery.
(B) Includes work done at Sydenham Children's Hospital before closure.
(C) Includes 1564 FCE's in oral surgery.

SOUTH WEST SECTOR

Hospital	Number of Births 1991	Number of Paediatric Medical FCE's (1) 1991/92 Code 420	Number of Tertiary Specialty FCE's (2) 1991/92	Total FCE's Children 1991/2 All Codes	Number of Consultants/ Professors Named	Average Length of Stay Comparison (3)
Royal Marsden (Sutton)			793	793	2	3.94/4.00
St. Helier/ Queen Mary's Carshalton	3756	4173	1586	9185	Not Known	QMC 2.84/3.13 St.H 4.28/2.86
Queen Mary's Roehampton	1690	1094	825	2924	Not Known	2.75/2.90
St. George's	2885	3628	980	6361	6	3.32/2.90
Atkinson Morley's	–	–	221	221		
Kingston	2538	2578				

(1) This information may include well babies

(2) Tertiary Specialty FCE's Specialty Codes: 150, 110, 170, 171, 301, 302, 303, 320, 340, 350, 361, 370, 400, 421, 800, 823, 830

(3) The first figures gives the average length of stay in the hospital in days for all paediatric FCE's. The second gives the comparison against all DRG codes taken into account on the database.

ANALYSIS OF INPATIENT PRICES IN TEN LONDON HOSPITALS

	A BLK £	A ECR £	(1, 2) B BLK £	(1, 2) B ECR £	C BLK £	C ECR £	(2) D BLK £	(2) D ECR £	(2) E BLK £	(2) E ECR £	F BLK £	F ECR £	G BLK £	G ECR £	H BLK £	H ECR £	(3) I BLK £	(3) I ECR £	(2, 4) J BLK £	(2, 4) J ECR £
Paediatric Medical FCE	1342	2409	938	938	-	744	1173	1093	825	-	519	-	-	-	1054	-	1450	1450	-	-
Neonatal Intensive Care	9457	(5) 13597	-	(6) 818	7759													(6) 600		(6) 639
Cardiac									(7) 3125				2908	1176						
Surgery (Emergency)	1430	2549					1245	1087	1822				2374		1159					
Surgery (Elective)	1430	1961					949	819					2374		1159					
Specialist Surgery (Emergency)							1728	1686												
Specialist Surgery (Elective)							1117	1062												
CAPD									3278								(8) 13650			

KEY: Blk = Block contract   ECR = Extra contractual referral

Notes:

1. Net of SIFT(R)
2. Price banding in operation
3. Adult and childrens prices the same
4. NICU high dependancy and special care charged per day

5. Up to fourteen days - thereafter charged per day
6. Price per day
7. Procedure pricing in operation
8. £5,250 if GP prescribes fluids

All prices exclusive of capital charges except Hospital D

LIST OF SUBMISSIONS TO REVIEW GROUP

(EXCLUDING HOSPITALS, COMMUNITY UNITS AND

HEALTH AUTHORITIES)

Charitable or Voluntary Organisations

The Retinoblastoma Society

The National Children's Bureau

The Leukaemia Care Society

The Child Growth Foundation

The Council for Disabled Children

Crohns in Childhood

Action for Sick Children

The British Kidney Patients Association

The Royal National Institute for the Blind

Sickle Cell Anaemia Relief (SCAR)

The Sick Children's Trust (Home from Home Appeal)

Steps - National Association for Children with Congenital Abnormalities of the Lower Limbs

The Save the Children Fund

The Malcolm Sargent Cancer Fund for Children

Child Accident Prevention Trust

National Children's Homes

Westminster Hospitals Development Fund (Mr A Meyer)

BACUP

The Cancer and Leukaemia in Childhood Trust (CLCT)

Imperial Cancer Research Fund, Professor J S Malpas

Community Health Councils

Greenwich Community Health Council

South East Kent Community Health Council

Tower Hamlets Community Health Council

City and Hackney Community Health Council

Professional Organisations and Individuals

Paediatric and Neonatal Surgery in South East London (Miss E H Dykes and others)

The Hospitals for Sick Children and Institute of Child Health (Joint R&D submission)

Dr A Woo, Consultant Rheumatology CRC

Dr N R Bennett, Chairman, Paediatric Intensive Care Society

Professor M Lewin, St Mary's Hospital, Medical School

Dr J A Sills, re children's rheumatology, Alder Hey Children's Hospital

Dr Owen Hanmer, Chairman, North East Thames Paediatric Advisory Committee

Dr P Jaffe, Chairman, North West Thames Advisory Committee

Dr A Ruben, BPMF, (SE Thames)

College of Ophthalmologists

British Paediatric Neurology Association

Professor J M Chessells: on behalf on Paediatric Oncologists in the Thames Regions

British Society of Paediatric Gastroenterology and Nutrition

British Paediatric Association

British Paediatric Cardiology Association

British Association of Paedatric Surgeons

Paediatric Intensive Care Society

British Paediatric Endocrinology Association

British Paediatric Respiratory Group

Royal College of Physicians

Paediatric Haematology Forum

The Royal College of Surgeons of England

Trade's Union Congress

The British Association of Urological Surgeons

Dr D S Arthur on behalf of the Association of Paediatric Anaesthetists

The Medical Research Council

The Royal College of Radiologists

Action for Sick Children

Mr E Hurst and others re paediatric oncology services in London

The United Kingdom Children's Cancer Study Group

The British Orthopaedic Association

The British Association of Plastic Surgeons

The Royal College of Nursing

The College of Occupational Therapists

Professor O B Eden, Professor of Paediatric Oncology, The Barts NHS Trust

Professor Brent Taylor, Professor of Community Child Health, The Royal Free Hospital

Dr T Stanton, The Secretariat for London Local Medical Committees

Dr A F Williams, re metabolic disease, St George's Hospital

Mr K Holmes, on behalf of Paediatric Surgeons in South West Thames

Dr M Bellman, North East RHAs, Community Paediatrician Group

Dr J E Hammond, Regional Adviser in Paediatrics, SWTRHA

Dr J F Price, Convenor, British Paediatric Respiratory Group

Professor Sir Colin Dollery, Pro-Vice Chancellor for Medicine and Dentistry, University of London

The Royal Pharmaceutical Society of Great Britain

Professor Levin, Professor of Paediatrics, St Mary's Hospital Medical School

The Society of Public Health

Mr B C Sommerlad: on behalf of a group of North East Thames Specialist Surgeons

Dr A Harris, Director of Clinical Policy and Research, Lewisham, Southwark annd Lambeth FHSA

The Royal College of Pathologists

Professor Graham Zellick, Principal, Queen Mary and Westfield College, Chair of London

C N Hudson, The London Hospital Medical College, Joint Academic Unit of Obstetrics, Gynaecology and Reproductive Physiology

Professor L Spitz, Nuffield Professor of Paediatric Surgery, Institute of Child Health

Mr N Madden, Consultant Paediatrician Surgeon, Chelsea and Westminster Hospital

The Chartered Society of Physiotherapy

The Royal College of Surgeons

Professor A W Craft, UK Children's Cancer Study Group

Dr A Vellodi, Riverside Health

Consultant Paediatric Intensivists - Great Ormond Street, St George's, St Mary's and Guy's,

Dr S A McKenzie, Consultant Paediatrician

Professor A P Mowat, Paediatric Hepatologist, King's Healthcare

Professor J A Walker-Smith, Professor of Paediatric Gastroenterology, Queen Elizabeth Hospital, Hackney

Professor C B S Wood, Joint Academic Department of Child Health, Queen Elizabeth Hospital, Hackney

Professor A R Nicol, Professor of Child Psychiatry, Royal College of Psychiatrists

Professor C Chantler, Principal, UMDS

Professor M Bobrow, Prince Philip Professor of Paediatric Research, UMDS

Professor C H Rodeck, Department of Obstetrics and Gynaecology, University College London Medical School

Professor K E Davies, Director of Research, Medical Research Centre, Hammersmith Hospital

Professor A Aynsley-Green, Nuffield Professor of Child Health, Institute of Child Health

Professor Sir Michael Rutter, Department of Child and Adolescent Psychiatry

Mr M L Rigby, Director of Paediatrics, Royal Brompton National Heart and Lung Hospital

Dr H B Valman, Clinical Director, Northwick Park Hospital

Mr G Davies, Consultant/Senior Lecturer in Child Health, St George's Medical School

Dr R J Postlethwaite, Consultant Paediatric Nephrologist/Secretary BAPN

Dr S J Chapman on behalf of South West Thames Regional Paediatricians

Royal College of Anaesthetists

British Medical Association

Dr S C Davies, Consultant Haeamtologist, Central Middlesex Hospital

Professor P Richards, Dean, St Mary's Hospital Medical School

Dr P J Flemming, Chairman BPA Working Party Paediatric Intensive Care

Independent Hospitals

The Independent Healthcare Association

BIBLIOGRAPHY

Paediatric Nephrology in the Nineties, The British Association for Paediatric Nephrology, 1992

London Health Care 2010 - Changing the Future of Services in the Capital and Working Papers 1-11, The King's Fund London Initiative, 1992

Parents Staying Overnight in Hospital with their Children, British Paediatric Association, National Association for the Welfare of Children in Hospital, National Association of Health Authorities, Royal College of Nursing, 1988

Just for the Day, Rosemary Thornes on behalf of Caring for Children in the Health Service, 1991

Paediatric Medical Staffing for the 1990's, The British Paediatric Association, April 1991

Access to and Availability of Specialist Services, Clinical Standards Advisory Group, March 1993

Neonatal Intensive Care, Clinical Standards Advisory Group, March 1993

London Postgraduate Hospitals' Comparative Costing Study, CASPE, 1993

Towards a Combined Child Health Service, British Paediatric Association, November 1991

Management Models in Established Combined or Integrated Child Health Services, British Paediatric Association, March 1992

Community Child Health Services - An Information Base for Purchasers, British Paediatric Association, February 1992

Guidance on Operation of Notification Arrangements for Tertiary Extra-Contractual Referrals HSG(93)8, NHS Management Executive, February 1993

Estate Information, NHS Estates, March 1993

Quality Management for Children - Play in Hospital, Christine Hogg on behalf of Play in Hospital Liaison Committee, 1990

Guidelines on the Management of Head Injuries in Childhood, Report of a Working Party of The British Paediatric Association and British Association of Paediatric Surgeons Joint Standing Committee on Childhood Accidents, August 1991

The Organisation of Services for Children with Diabetes in the United Kingdom, Report of a British Paediatric Association Working Party, August 1989

Report of the Joint Working Party on Liver Transplantation in Children, British Paediatric Association and British Association of Paediatric Surgeons, April 1986

Neurophysiological Services for Children in the United Kingdom, Report of a British Paediatric Association, British Paediatric Neurology Association and Association of British Clinical Neurophysiologists, January 1989

Outcome Measurements for Child Health, British Paediatric Association, November 1992

Report of the Joint Working Party on Medical Services for Children, Dr A W Macara, Joint Working Party of Medical Services for Children, November 1992

Childhood Leukaemia - Access to and Availability of Specialist Services, Clinical Standards Advisory Group, February 1993

Cystic Fibrosis - Access to and Availability of Specialist Services, Clinical Standards Advisory Group, February 1993

Transfer of Infants and Children for Surgery, British Paediatric Association, 1993

Workload of Consultant Paediatricians, Joint Guidelines of the British Medical Association, British Paediatric Association and Paediatric Committees of the Royal Colleges of Physicians of London and Edinburgh and of the Royal College of Physicians and Surgeons of Glasgow, September 1990

8.6.93

Printed in the United Kingdom for HMSO.
Dd.296539, 6/93, C35, 3396/4, 5673, 249611.